A Study into Infant Mental Health

This book is a study of infant mental health which blends knowledge and understanding from three perspectives: international research, theory, and intervention. The volume increases awareness of the significance of infant mental health, adding to the growing body of literature on influences upon lifestyles, communities, society, and attainment.

The significance of mental health to development has come to the fore in recent years and research in neuroscience is used to explore, and to understand the complexities of the human brain. Each infant is exposed to unique influences before and after birth. Neuroscience, genetics, adverse childhood experiences, and personalities feature in the chapters as mitigating factors to attainment. Exemplars create a bridge between research and implementation of recommendations, and illustrate the myriad of influences and permutations that can enhance or hinder development. This book discusses internal influences from an infant's biological make-up, alongside the circumstances and relationships within a family unit, as understanding these key aspects is integral to promotion of each infant's life chances. The volume concludes by considering future approaches to nurturing infant mental health.

Carefully designed to stimulate discussion and professional inquiry, this volume is an invaluable resource for researchers, academics, and scholars with an interest in infant mental health.

Hazel G. Whitters is a practitioner-researcher who works in an early years service in Glasgow, Scotland. Interests include the professional–parent relationship, therapeutic play, and infant mental health.

Advances in Mental Health Research

A Study into Infant Mental Health

Drawing together Perspectives of
International Research, Theory, and
Practical Intervention

Hazel G. Whitters

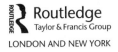

Routledge
Taylor & Francis Group
LONDON AND NEW YORK

Designed cover image: © Getty Images

First published 2023
by Routledge
4 Park Square, Milton Park, Abingdon, Oxon OX14 4RN

and by Routledge
605 Third Avenue, New York, NY 10158

Routledge is an imprint of the Taylor & Francis Group, an informa business

British Library Cataloguing-in-Publication Data
A catalogue record for this book is available from the British Library

ISBN: 978-1-032-41441-6 (hbk)
ISBN: 978-1-032-41445-4 (pbk)
ISBN: 978-1-003-35810-7 (ebk)

DOI: 10.4324/9781003358107

Typeset in Times New Roman
by Taylor & Francis Books

I dedicate this book to children, parents, and carers throughout the world. Nurturing the next generation is key to attainment for all within happy, fulfilling lives. I include a dedication to my husband John whose continuous support and encouragement has enabled me to achieve. Thank you.

Contents

Preface

This book is a monograph that presents knowledge and understanding of infant mental health from the three perspectives of research, theory, and intervention. I hope that this monograph will stimulate discussion and professional inquiry from scholars and researchers. I have worked for 40 years in childcare and education, and in the past 12 years I have undertaken research and training in infant mental health. The key to an infant's independent learning is transformation of his inner working model.

This monograph aims to engage readers by contributing to the knowledge base that informs issues pertaining to this field of study. Current and past research from international sources is used to increase a reader's understanding of mental-health issues in young children with an emphasis on neural development and the impact of adversities. Participants in these studies have experienced negative influences upon development and include minority groups. A deeper understanding of neuroscience and environmental impact is gained by contextualising research findings within daily lifestyles.

Knowledge is weak as a single entity but rich if accompanied by understanding which can influence strategy and, ultimately, implementation of intervention. I feel passionately that learning and professional development should be shared with others to generate discussion, investigation, and to increase expertise in the field of infant mental health.

This book discusses the attainment gap by accessing research on high ability, additional learning needs, and developmental norms. The current focus upon attainment is contextualised by reference to the COVID-19 pandemic. COVID-19 has presented a new multilayered adversity and prompted professionals to seek out knowledge and to reflect upon pertinent issues. The lockdown periods narrowed the daily world of the workforce but increased opportunities and time for research and professional development. Infant mental-health teams are being established throughout the world to target this area of need.

The pandemic has resulted in unpredicted influences upon mental health in adults, children, and infants. The book describes how children are presenting in services with unusual demonstration of trauma which is emerging within research as associated with social and emotional isolation, and parents' anxieties.

Knowledge and understanding of these aspects feature in studies throughout the world, and findings will continue to be published over the coming months and years.

I feel that this is an opportune time to write a monograph in response to these issues. The book is designed to increase awareness of the significance of infant mental health through presentation of research, theory, and intervention, and to add to the growing body of literature on influences upon lifestyles, communities, society, and attainment. This book is primarily aimed at scholars in the disciplines of health, education, social work, and family therapy.

1 Infant mental health

Chapter 1 commences by considering the meaning of infant mental health and by using the definition of Zeanah and Zeanah (2019) to refer to the period of pre-birth to five years throughout the manuscript. This chapter provides an explanation of infant mental health and detailed description of the neurobiological changes that occur pre-birth and post-birth. Research in the field of neuroscience (Dismukes et al., 2019) has greatly increased understanding of brain development. The physiological impact of adversities upon neural connections is discussed, for example, disorganised attachment at the age of one year is regarded as a predictor of psychopathology in adolescence (Cassidy & Mohr, 2001). Practice examples provide narratives to illustrate research findings. Genetics and environmental circumstances are identified as influential in contexts of experience-dependent and experience-expectant stages of development. Stress is described from a neural and behavioural perspective which includes the short- or long-term effects from normal, tolerable, and toxic stress upon an infant and parent (Shonkoff et al., 2021). Formal and informal interventions are highlighted as valuable responses to infant mental-health issues which are founded upon secure attachment relationships.

Understanding infant mental health

The terms "infant mental health" and "child" in this book refer to the period from pre-birth to five years as used by Zeanah and Zeanah (2019). Other organisations refer to infant mental health as encompassing slightly different timescales within early childhood. The Scottish Perinatal Mental Health Curricular Framework describes the perinatal period as pregnancy, childbirth, and the first 12 months of childhood (NHS Education for Scotland, 2019). The emotional aspect of infant mental health, in accordance with the framework, links to the attachment relationship from birth which has long-term implications throughout the lifespan. This publication also presents stages of infant mental health which include 3–5 years. The Infant Mental Health Competency Framework is targeted towards professionals who work with parents and infants from pregnancy to the second year of life (Association of Infant Mental Health, UK, 2021). In 2000, a researcher published an article

DOI: 10.4324/9781003358107-1

that focused upon the role, responsibilities, and characteristics of the infant mental-health specialist. The specialism related to working with parents and children from birth to three years of age (Weatherston, 2000).

Despite slight variation in age groups which are associated with the term "infant", or "child", these authors universally define infant mental health as a young child's capacity for social and emotional development. Social and emotional development are intertwined, and one is dependent upon the other. In 2019, the concept of infant mental health was broadened to include positive cognitive development by NHS Education for Scotland (2019). Certain conditions are necessary to support these aspects of human development to mature. Trevarthan and Aitken (2001) inserted context and rationale to the study of mental health in young children by stating that it created a foundation for interpersonal needs throughout the lifespan. This chapter explores these issues in the perinatal and antenatal periods.

Perinatal mental health has recently come to the forefront of practice in health disciplines as a significant aspect of care and education from birth to five years. A baby's mental health is also influenced before birth. The perinatal stage is regarded from the pre-birth period up to one year post-birth. Pregnancy, childbirth, and the first year of life are periods when intervention can make positive changes to the mental health of a mother and her infant. Extended family members can also be affected by maternal and infant mental-health issues. Research has indicated that postnatal depression which is not treated can have a negative impact upon the operational daily functioning of a family unit (Balbernie, 2013).

In the earliest stage of life, a young child's emotions are led by physical needs relating to survival. At birth, a baby is exposed to a multitude of sensory stimuli. His instinct is not to explore but to seek comfort. His instinct is not to learn but to gain protection in this new world in which he cannot differentiate between danger and safety. His needs are based upon physical survival, and emotions lead his body to a state of alert by prioritising these goals. The newborn has only one familiar contact within the initial moments of entry to the world. Nurture by his mother is welcomed by the tiny baby as her voice is recognisable from his pre-birth experiences, and over time her warmth and smell represent a circle of security. This circle embraces the infant physically and emotionally.

These potent statements elevate and prioritise infant mental health within the context of childcare and education services. During the past twenty years the concept of mental health has received attention from researchers, and governments, due to an increase in comprehension of the long-term impact upon the individual and society. In the United Kingdom, one in five children are diagnosed with an emotional behavioural disorder which is experienced as internal trauma and exhibited externally through behaviour. Disorganised attachment at the age of one year is regarded as a predictor of psychopathology in adolescence (Cassidy & Mohr, 2001).

Many countries have focused upon exploring and supporting mental health in infants. For example, in Scotland a multidisciplinary group of professionals compiled the Perinatal Mental Health Curricular Framework which reflects learning levels for the professional, as depicted within the NES Transforming Psychological Trauma Network (NHS Education for Scotland, 2019). These levels of continuous professional development are constructed in an incremental way and describe four stages of knowledge, understanding, and practical skill in the field of infant mental health: informed, skilled, enhanced, and specialist. It is interesting that the four levels transcend many different roles and responsibilities in disciplines throughout care and education fields. The rationale for this broad spectrum gives significance to multidisciplinary roles in a context of mental-health knowledge and practical skill.

Pre-birth and post-birth

Antenatal is termed from birth onwards so there is an overlap of time in which the two descriptors of perinatal and antenatal can be applied to the first 12 months of childhood. A mother is a baby's host before birth so it is inevitable that her mental health will impact upon the baby's well-being during the gestation months. Figures were published by NHS England in May 2021 that recorded the number of women who accessed perinatal mental health services in 2019–2020. This coincided with lockdown periods of the COVID-19 pandemic, and the figure of 4.6 per cent of total births was slightly above the predicted level of 4.5 per cent. The figure 4.6 per cent equates to 30,625 women.

Zeanah and Zeanah (2019) describe mental health in a context of capacity; therefore, targeting support to a mother *during* pregnancy is an essential context for intervention by services. The ultimate aim is to increase the infant's capacity for good mental health throughout his life. The National Centre for Infant and Early Childhood Health Policy, in America, identified three levels of intervention: universal and preventative services, focused services, and tertiary intervention service (Zeanah et al., 2005). This report referred to mitigating factors as relating to the environment, infant, parent or carer, and the adult–child relationship. Relationships are promoted as the most important aspect of any parenting programme or informal intervention.

Pregnancy is a time of change, physically and emotionally. It is a period in which a woman and her partner acquire different roles and responsibilities in the creation of a new life, and adaptation of a family home, and lifestyle. The research of Slade and Sadler (2019) emphasised influences from the conception route to the parents' emotional adaptation. Factors related to a pregnancy being assisted or non-assisted, and planned or unexpected. The pathway towards, and during pregnancy, affects both parents' conscious and unconscious experiences and their reactions to the early stages of parenthood.

It has been shown that a mother's brain has an increase in growth and development of social and emotional connections preceding and following birth. The state of pregnancy prepares the mother's neural networks for mentalisation and a nurturing capacity that supports an infant's socio-emotional development. The neural networks which are activated throughout pregnancy include the oxytocin system relating to attachment and bonding, the hypothalamic–pituitary–adrenal axis to regulate stress and respond to danger, and the dopaminergic centre as the area of the brain that activates pleasure experiences (Slade & Sadler, 2019). Examples of pre-natal stress include socio-economic adversity, domestic or community violence, isolation within an environment or culture of a community, and mental-health issues. The emotional and physical status of a mother will impact directly or indirectly upon her baby, pre-birth and post-birth.

Neural development

Research in the field of neuroscience (Dismukes et al., 2019) has greatly increased understanding of brain development and portrays the composition of a neuron that has a **cell body, axon**, and **dendrites**. Brain growth is complex, and dependent upon influences between physiological, emotional, and genetic characteristics of an infant. An outcome is the creation of links between neurons. The space between neurons is termed **synaptic cleft**, and the process of connection is **synaptogenesis**.

It is fascinating to read that the branching between dendrites occurs when the neuron nucleus is full, which means that it has accumulated its maximum complement of electrical inputs. At this stage electrical inputs will continue to be received but travel down the axon, cross the synaptic cleft through neurotransmitters, and branch out to different dendrites. These dendrites lead to more neurons, and neural connections are established.

Questions emerge from reading about brain processes, for example, does the neuron nucleus release all the electrical outputs together at the point of maximum capacity? Perhaps the release occurs in minuscule levels for output to the axon, in tandem with further input of electrical impulses. Reaching capacity may be the catalyst for this process to be initiated. I reflect upon my thoughts on potential patterns or timed sequences in the release, and uptake of electrical charges, and consider if I can relate this neural process to practice knowledge. It is important that new learning which contains challenging issues is retained and can be applied in linking research to daily practice.

The axons are well protected by insulation in the form of myelin. The myelin allows the electrical inputs to travel very quickly along the axons to cross the space of the synaptic cleft. Neural circuits which are created throughout this process are termed synaptic transmission. Over time, pruning takes place of synapses which are not being used, or less actively used than others. It seems that the myelination process protects the circuits from being pruned.

These processes are often represented in training for practice by the use of cartoon symbols and sequences that demonstrate interdependency of components. An animation medium can promote understanding of these events in a straightforward, predictable, and simplistic way. It is also essential that practitioners appreciate the intricacies of brain development, and the myriad of mitigating factors. It is a fascinating topic to study which imposes respect and worthiness to the role of an early years practitioner. I feel that knowledge of neural processes instils a sense of wonder, and awe as understanding of the complexities are gained.

From a practical perspective, a lack of nurturing conditions, or direct influences from adversities can prevent the neuron nucleus from reaching its capacity. These barriers are described in practice as hindering or halting achievement of potential. Subsequent branching and links between dendrites and further neurons will not take place. This information gives stark realisation of the significance of early intervention work to construction of the brain's architecture that affects the baby throughout his lifespan.

Classification of the nervous system by functionality presents a visual picture of the internal layout and workings of the neural space. Mechanisms for basic life functions are tucked safely in the middle of the brain, surrounded by the cortex which supports the higher-level functioning of human beings. The frontal, parietal, occipital, and temporal cortex lobes have essential roles to play in the infant's interpretation of the world which is based on sensory experience and communication with others.

The 27th day after conception is obviously a significant milestone in pregnancy due to formation of the neural tube which is the foundation for the brain and spinal cord. It is interesting that one reason for significant brain growth *after* birth is to ensure a safe birth passage. The small brain is protected from damage during the birthing process and subsequently grows rapidly in the early stages of childhood. A baby's brain increases in weight by 2.5 times from birth to 12 months of age. Neural development in such a short period is influenced by environmental conditions, internal well-being, and the infant–primary carer relationship. The first year of life is a sensitive period of learning for the mother and child thus presenting an optimum opportunity for early intervention.

Adversities and stress responses

Research has indicated that life experiences can have a positive effect on creating and consolidating the connections between neurons (Gerhardt, 2004). Bowlby (1979) describes reconfiguration of the inner working model as the processes occur and the neural connections extend and create branches to adjoining cells. An image is gained of foetal neurons busily connecting and ensuring viability through the establishment of a framework for bodily functions, between 5 and 9 months of pregnancy. This stage of development encompasses information that health professionals can easily share with expectant parents, and initiate responsibility for the well-being of their unborn child.

Toxic stress is defined by the enduring time and impact upon the individual's biological responses and interlinked emotional consequences. The toxicity results from interactions between environmental influences, personal experiences, genetic predisposition, and developmental timing (Shonkoff et al., 2021). Stress can have a toxic impact during the same period of development in which an infant is known to be affected by specific bacterial species. The bacteria are described as colonising the newborn baby's intestines, following influences from maternal transmission and environmental exposure, and can result in a lifelong impact upon immune functions. Adversities which are experienced in the perinatal period can increase the infant's vulnerability to physiological and psychosocial stressors thereafter.

Shonkoff et al. (2021) presented evidence that indicated that the prevalent biological response to early adversity is a predisposition to a chronic pro-inflammatory phenotype. There are associations with conditions such as cardiovascular disease, chronic obstructive pulmonary disease, autoimmune disease, and depression. The authors suggest targeted intervention to specific minority groups within the earliest years to promote equality in health and well-being, and to increase opportunities for lifelong achievement. The optimum intervention is preventative and proactive: reduction of the impact from toxic stress, in addition to measures that aim to increase the child's resilience and promote educational attainment.

The two systems for responding to stress are the sympathomedullary (SAM) system, and the hypothalmic–pituitary–adrenal (HPA) axis. It was useful for my own practice to learn that the hormone adrenalin, as a regulator of cell/organ activity, can take up to 20 minutes to course around the body through the bloodstream (Berens & Nelson, 2019). However, an emergency "universal energy store" of adenosine triphosphate (ATP) is situated within muscles to enable an immediate response to threat by releasing chemical energy that triggers a physical reaction. In reality, an infant can respond by moving away from a negative influence, and his body undergoes physiological changes to support this reaction to adversity. The external stress results in internal changes as epinephrine (adrenalin) increases circulation and breathing rates and releases glycogen throughout the body. The body makes this response based upon rapid assessment of the immediacy of a threat.

Early stages of development

Cortical inhibitory control commences between 2 and 4 months of age. Mothers and carers notice subtle changes in the baby's behaviour and his emotions during this time. For example, the neonatal reflexes subside, and sleep–wake cycles can be recognised. These patterns of behaviour within routines are influenced by cultural parenting practices. Parents gain a growing awareness of their baby's needs and personalities, and the baby begins to demonstrate consistency in his reactions and actions in response to common daily events. His lifestyle becomes immersed within a family culture. At this stage, parents are encouraged by health workers and practitioners to establish routines that suit the baby's emerging needs. Changes can occur rapidly as the infant gains an awareness of his proximal environment in addition to the influences from his primary carers.

At 9 or 10 months, the baby uses memory and goal-directed behaviour in his responses to stimulation, as opposed to response tendencies which was the term applied by Thompson (1991). An attentive carer adapts the proximal environment to reflect the baby's emerging personality and needs, and his learning processes are stimulated and activated by these increasing opportunities. Over time, the infant perceives the circle of security which is provided by his secure attachment relationship with a primary carer. This circle is represented physically and emotionally, and it enables the infant to demonstrate his preferences, interests, and emotional or physical reaction to his lifestyle. An infant actively seeks out experiences that match his personality and developmental needs from birth. The initial 12 months of life are a significant period for learning, and the baby should be supported by carers to maintain good health for genetic potential in the neural connections to be fulfilled. A stimulating and safe environment in which to learn about the world is essential at home and within services.

Shonkoff et al. (2021) presents an interactive gene–environment–time framework. The framework encompasses several aspects which are influential to development. This approach to understanding infant brain development reflects the influences from an infant's adaptation to different contexts, his immune system, metabolic regulation, and the plasticity of his neural connections. Examples of change can be detected in systemic inflammation and insulin responsivity. Variation in sensitivity to these influences is a significant factor, particularly among siblings, and it is influenced by personality in addition to genetic composition of the body. The conclusion of this research study explains that gaining understanding of the interplay between preventative, and responsive intervention, is key to determining effective primary health care in early childhood. A responsive adult, who interacts with an infant in a context of a secure attachment relationship, has an invaluable role in overcoming or preventing negative impact upon development in the earliest years.

Shonkoff et al. (2021) also apply the term "relationship-focused coaching" as a means of supporting primary carers to create effective relationships with an infant. Care which is given in a context of a positive relationship compliments the implementation of preventative, and resilience measures in adversity. These authors highlight the promotion of secure attachment as a response to perinatal depression. Findings from this particular research study identified targeted interventions as the promotion of male caregiver interactions and home-visiting programmes. Additional measures included limiting the use of media screen time for parent, and child, and increasing literacy in a context of adult–child book interactions. Reduction of economic stress can also increase the capacity of an adult to participate in caregiving activities with an infant. Examples of useful daily activities are consistent and predictable routines that focus upon feeding, resting, and play. Brain development responds positively to this model of a caring environment.

Box 1.1 Example from practice

Jake was referred to our service by his health visitor. *Infant mental health due to trauma of home circumstances.* This broad referral criteria presented little information excepting a young child who was suffering emotionally, cognitively, and physically, as affected by indeterminate influences.

At induction day, Dad stood at the back door waiting patiently as I rushed down the long corridor to welcome the family. It was raining, a wet cold January shower. Dad's face mask made his voice sound muffled and devoid of emotion. I could not see Jake. I quickly introduced myself to Dad and ushered him into the service. The bright fluorescent lights and blast of heat emanating from the service was stark contrast to the inclement weather. Behind Dad I spotted Jake. A small slim child of three years who was wearing a yellow jacket with a hood tightly pulled under his chin. My greeting was directed towards this little child's eyes as he peeked out from under the raindrops.

We entered a meeting room which released a scent of antibacterial cleaning products. I noticed that Jake wrinkled his nose as he was encompassed by the new environment. Dad perched on the edge of a settee and faced me silently as he pulled the little boy onto his knee. Dad loosened his son's outer clothing and began to talk. Mother had a difficult birth, memories of losing a previous baby, diabetes during pregnancy, postnatal depression, work stopped due to COVID-19 lockdowns, lack of money, cold house, always using food bank – Mum can't leave the house. This final comment encapsulated the difficulties faced by the family within a myriad of influences that could be fitted easily into a bio-ecological framework of human development.

I thanked this family for attending our service. I showed photographs of our playrooms and garden areas – unfortunately out of bounds to parents during this pandemic. Jake pointed to the pictures, and Dad described the scene to his son. At this point I had observed a healthy dad and son who appeared to have an attachment relationship that involved comfortable physical contact and responsive interaction, albeit within this stark environment of a cleaned-down meeting room. Suddenly Jake made a loud growling noise, threw his two arms back against his dad, and slid to the floor. His wet jacket made this slide quick and easy, and the little boy gave me direct eye contact as he leaned forward to spit. I quietly said to Dad, "Jake is showing us that he is tired of talking and he just wants to play, and to learn."

The care plan for this family had commenced through attendance at nursery. Each adversity, as cited by Dad, had an influence upon the adults and children and required sensitive exploration and actions to minimise the effect. Each influence conjoined with others to create an accumulative negative impact upon the family's well-being. Jake's behaviour, delayed development, and aggressive outbursts represented this little three-year-old's vivid reactions to his family circumstances, daily challenges from the pandemic, his expressions of need, and desire to have his interests met. Behaviour is language, the original communication media of human beings, and Jake's expression of his emotions in the context of adverse childhood experiences.

Theory and infant mental health

The World Association of Infant Mental Health (WAIMH, 2000), and the Zero to Three taskforce (2001) present clear descriptors of infant mental health. The former emphasises an active response by adults in promotion of an infant's mental health which is equated with optimal development for the whole family. The latter presents an infant's developing social and emotional capacity which enables his learning and development to progress. Reference is made to the bio-ecological systems theory (Bronfenbrenner, 1979; Bronfenbrenner & Morris, 2006) on which practice models and curricular guidance are based. This framework represents the multilayered and multidirectional influences upon development of a human being.

Practitioners learn about developmental milestones in relation to a child's age during undergraduate study. Frameworks of normative development provide a means to identify delay. The early childhood ecosystem, as termed by Shonkoff et al. (2021), presents understanding of external influences upon development. Post-qualification, it is important that this knowledge is maintained to provide a framework for identification and response to temporary or long-term additional support for learning needs. Temporary needs may result from a change of home circumstances, for example, different carers, accommodation, or lifestyle of parents. The mantra that I have learned over a 40-year career in services is that there is a solution to every problem, and life can be good, life can be fulfilling, and happiness is achievable by every individual and family.

Sloan and Donnelly (2021) recently conducted research on perinatal mental health in the Glasgow area of central Scotland. The focus was an investigatory study on factors that inhibited or protected the mental health of expectant mothers. The projected outcome was to map service provision and contribute to an improvement plan for the entire city. This research was conducted as the COVID-19 pandemic was emerging across the United Kingdom, and throughout the world. Findings identified a range of personal and socio-economic factors that the 200 participants identified as impacting upon mental health. Poverty, housing, childcare, and stigma associated with perception of failure in the parenting role were recurrent issues in the data. The youth of parents, ethnic origin, and traumatic experiences were additional factors that participants expressed as affecting mental health during pregnancy. Interestingly, the study revealed provision for severe perinatal health in this city but lack of services that offered early intervention or prevention in a context of "mild to moderate" mental-health problems, as defined within this research. Accessible community services were recommended by the research team in addition to peer support from family, friends, and services.

Bronfenbrenner (2005) presented influences in pictorial form as the bio-ecological systems of human development. Concentric circles indicate potential bidirectional links between four main systems with the infant at the centre:

1   The **microsystem** refers to influences from structure, processes, and relationships closest to the child, for example, family unit and services. The microsystem also represents family culture, which may be influenced by religion, nationality, community, or parental choices.
2   The **mesosystem** refers to influences from processes that bridge the settings in which the infant is involved, for example, the nursery–home links. This source of impact is significant for the early years workforce.
3   The **exosystem** refers to indirect influences between settings, for example, changes to a parent's workplace may affect attendance patterns at nursery.
4   The **macrosystem** refers to influences that affect all systems through policy, procedures, and legislation. The macrosystem encompasses community and societal expectations.

Bronfenbrenner also refers to time as an important consideration within a context of development. Influences and their impact upon a family change over time, and certainly the infant's responses will alter as he matures. The knowledge and understanding within his inner working model increases, and it is refined by retaining salient points that relate to personal characteristics and genetic disposition. The developing infant gains more options as his experiences and capacity to make positive personal and social choices increase.

Epigenetics

Epigenetics is a familiar concept for researchers, and it indicates links between environmental influences and activation of genes by changes in the body before and after birth. Effective planning and implementation of learning opportunities relies on knowledge of each child's interests and needs in a context of child-led pedagogy. The findings of Dismukes et al. (2019) indicated five important points regarding epigenetics.

1   Epigenetics entails a set of interactive processes.
2   Development occurs within a reciprocal relationship between the environment and biology – before and after birth.

3 Environmental changes can affect interaction of these epigenetic processes.
4 Disruptions to development in infancy can result in long-term negative impact across the lifespan.
5 Brain plasticity can provide opportunities, or threats to development, as the neural connections reflect experiences which are positive *and* negative to the infant's well-being.

Characteristics of an individual are sourced to two sets of influences (Dismukes et al., 2019):

1 Genes – 50–80 per cent influence.
2 Environment – 20–50 per cent influence.

These figures portray a broad range and, most importantly, the knowledge that characteristics are informed by activation of genes and interaction with environmental influences. The genotype or genetic make-up that affects a baby's physical characteristics is innate but greatly influenced pre-birth and post-birth. Additionally, temperament or phenotype can be affected negatively by a parent's lifestyle and reflected within the infant's interpretation and reaction to the world. Common examples of family adversities are parental drug or alcohol use, domestic violence, poverty, and isolation in a community.

In my experience, the physical presentation of an infant who is living in adversity can change markedly after he has been taken into kinship or foster care, even for short-term respite. Hair colouring can transform from low-nutritional grey to natural healthy pigment, weight and height are gained rapidly, sad eyes begin to shine with hope and motivation, and demonstration of the positive aspects of temperament are observable features that indicate good care. It is important that positive change is recorded in addition to negative as it clearly highlights the influential aspects of a previous home environment and pinpoints areas for intervention. Physical and mental well-being can activate an infant's motivation to seek out learning as opposed to maintaining his basic bodily functions within survival mode. This knowledge is gained through observation and assessment by a practitioner. Many countries use intervention to close the attainment gap in recognition of the impact of adversities. For example, my work is based in Glasgow city which is currently responding to the attainment gap in relation to poverty, and family learning is promoted as an effective strategy to change (Scottish Government, 2019).

Emotions and resilience

Resilience of an infant is apparent during his interactions and involvement with a learning environment. These features associated with development can be recorded within a matrix that indicates links between protective factors, adversities, vulnerability of the infant, and his resilience. National guidance, or recording scales, may highlight these issues and promote understanding of the impact from multiple adversities (Scottish Government, 2008; Laevers, 1994).

Fogel (1982) describes affective tolerance as the young child's ability and capacity to cope positively with stimulation which can lead to heightened excitement. This research study focused upon a period within the first 6 months of childhood prior to language development. New parents can learn to read their baby's emotional and attentional cues within this time of rapid change, for example, motivation, disinterest, fatigue, or overstimulation, and to respond with affective attunement (Stern, 1985). Affective attunement can be a catalyst to emotional regulation by an infant. Alternatively, lack of parental responsiveness can negatively affect the advent of the infant's emotional capacity, particularly in a context of adversities.

Thompson (1991) emphasised a link between emotional regulation in early childhood and the capacity of adults to self-regulate. Emotion is represented by behaviour and actions, and it is influenced by the ability and capacity to self-regulate. It is an important aspect of planning for practice that an infant is offered choices throughout daily routines to gain an awareness of his sense of self from an early age. Emotional processing is inherently linked to one's own needs, interests, and personality.

The phenomenon of "take-up" time is regularly observed in childhood and throughout formal learning circumstances of adulthood. Parents and practitioners may misinterpret the associated actions as disengagement. Young babies may turn away from excessive stimulation during reciprocal interaction, and research has shown an intake in sugar to the brain at this stage. It is recognised that primary-aged children require absorption time for the brain to retain knowledge, sometimes termed, "the 10 second rule" in education, and adult learners will swiftly look away from a lecturer as the brain assimilates information to gain understanding.

Creation of a foundation for these self-regulating strategies commences in the earliest years of life, and social referencing from adult to infant contributes to socialisation within a family, a community, and supports children to integrate within the wider world over time. The development of language increases capacity to self-regulate emotions. Language provides a universal forum for parents to discuss emotions, and prior experiences with children which enriches their comprehension of situations. Language also enables the child to gain symbolic recognition of his internal emotional state and to create links to influences in the external world.

The management of emotions is a contributory factor to effective learning. Processes include the child's ability and capacity to minimise negative emotions by transferring his attention to another area of learning. The foundation of emotional self-regulation commences at birth, and primary carers are influential in supporting this aspect of an infant's development. The adult's emotional responses to the infant are based upon family culture and beliefs which contribute to a role model. Another effect comes from the adult guiding the child towards a specific emotional response which may be led by implicit or explicit social rules.

The research findings by Thompson (1991) referred to the use of self-talk by a child and singing to oneself as a further strategy for self-regulation. Singing and self-talk can serve the purpose of blocking or reducing sensory intake, and these strategies can support a child to regain control of his emotional status, albeit for a few moments or longer. Self-regulation links to the child's personality, his perceived social status, and his desire to identify with a social group reaction, or to focus inwards to his own needs and preferences.

As this knowledge base increases then the child acquires emotional literacy and the ability to self-regulate his emotions, actions, and reactions. Over time, an understanding of pride and morality is influenced by cultural values and beliefs of the family, and potentially the local community or service setting. Attendance in services greatly enhances these processes by providing multiple opportunities for the child to experience and to understand emotional literacy. The child's comprehension of consequences, for example, the repercussions of displaying negative behaviour in a setting, demonstrates his integration and discrimination of social contexts and emotional parameters. As a child matures then he begins to associate emotional regulation and personal gain with a growing awareness of the negative impact from anger, fear, or frustration upon his desire to learn, and to achieve goals.

Young babies experience different internal states in relation to rage, fear, pain, loss, play, and care. Activation of a baby's emotions results in physiological change. Cortisol is released and influences behaviour and actions. These internal reactions contribute to the infant/child's developing sense of self over time. Emotions are deeply entwined with socialisation and expectations of feelings in relation to a family and community culture. An infant's interpretation of the world can be led by the primary carer's reaction or the role model of a practitioner. Babies may reflect the emotions of a parent which can be prohibitive of positive emotional development if the parent is suffering from short- or long-term mental-health issues. Young children's emotional literacy can be supported and the early stages of self-regulation initiated through sensitive care that supports up-regulation and promotes a pathway to down-regulation. Practice should respond to the child's personality and needs.

Thompson (1991) described a developmental stage that emerges around 36 months, termed meta-emotive understanding or knowledge of emotional processes. The young child has increasing capacity to recognise and to use strategies that are associated with self-regulation of emotions. He gains comprehension of conditions that lead to heightened emotions and the resultant sensory experiences, the reactions of other people in this context, and psychological processes. This study found that adults managed emotions by changing their surroundings and minimising or increasing direct influences upon their emotional responses. Alternatively, children's emotional self-regulation involved restriction of the stimuli which was usually at a sensory level.

A child may reduce sensory intake by covering eyes and ears to block the stimulatory input. The outcome is relative to the emotional stimulus being reduced rather than the emotion being regulated by the child. Additionally, a child may ignore circumstances of emotional arousal by turning away from the situation or turning towards a primary carer. A carer can support a child to interpret and to react positively to stimuli. For example, the sound of sirens of emergency vehicles or reverse horns on utility vehicles form a common backdrop to play within inner cities. Carers can support a child to gain understanding through linking to small-world play, showing a child the source of the sound from a window, and role-modelling interest and curiosity as opposed to fear and anxiety. Common occurrences within services or home environment present invaluable opportunities for development of self-regulation.

Experience-expectant and experience-dependent stages

I considered these findings in the context of my practice within a playroom for infants aged 0–2 years. Referrals for placement in a service give details of perceived stresses upon babies and children, for example, domestic violence, substance misuse, parents' additional support needs, and mental-health issues. Negative circumstances and assumption of positive influences may be presented within neatly compartmentalised sections of a referral form: adversity, protective factors, vulnerability, and resilience. However, the child's personality and his evolving sense of self are key aspects in his interpretation and reaction to influences. Siblings who attend the same service often demonstrate different reactions to adversities within the family home.

Experience-expectant and experience-dependent stages of development give clear representations of the responsibilities of carers. Experience-expectant is associated with support, which is given in a context of the normative pathways of development, for example, feeding and walking independently. These areas of development relate to neural connections that form after the infant has undergone a regular experience: a cry of hunger being rewarded by his mother's milk or a desire to walk being supported by a nurturing relationship and stimulating environment. This type of development is time-limited as it occurs within a critical period (Berens & Nelson, 2019).

In contrast, experience-dependent development is relative to personal experience and may occur in infancy and throughout the lifespan. Experience-dependent is the cultural influence upon synaptogenesis. Stimulation and development of the five senses requires exposure to light, sound, touch, smell, and a variety of tastes. Many children attend services in their early years of childhood on placements which are funded by governments. This funded strategic approach to education broadens the young child's exposure to learning opportunities. Research shows that experience-dependent learning is most effective during sensitive learning stages with a focus upon birth to 3 years (Centre for Excellence and Outcomes in Children and Young People's Services, 2010).

Berens and Nelson (2019) present an illustrative example of behaviour that may be influenced by development based upon experience-expectancy and experience-dependency. These authors describe the capacity of an infant to form attachment as being experience-expectant which occurs within the earliest stages of childhood. However, the quality of attachment reflects the personal experience-dependent learning opportunities which are offered to the infant by his primary carer.

At entry to a service, some children are vigilant, which is demonstrated by quick reactions and physical withdrawal from assumed sources of threat. The infant's perceived sources of threat include adults or peers breaching the personal space around his body, unexpected movements in his visual peripheries, and unidentifiable loud noises from outside the immediate setting. Nurturing and reassurance are offered to the infant by practitioners but may be rejected in the early stages of a relationship and interpreted as a potential threat. Physical and emotional contact which is given to the infant by a key worker may result in an increase in signs of his stress, for example, rapid heartbeat and perspiration. These physiological responses can appear as an overreaction by an infant within the caring and supportive context of a service.

Knowledge of physiological reactions will support comprehension of a practitioner in these circumstances and increase expertise in delivering responsive care to the infant's emotions. I have often encountered practitioners who do not fully understand trauma in childhood feeling rejected by an infant who creates a barrier to relationships. Practitioners in an early years service may not have access to the details of a family's circumstances. However, daily observations can provide invaluable information to support intervention in response to the infant's interpretation of his experiences.

The complex internal working of an infant in this context can result in exhaustion during and after these episodes. The practitioner presents a buffering relationship to minimise the effects but equally importantly by offering positive experiences within a child's world to reconfigure his inner working model and to use the secure attachment relationship for the optimum outcomes. Babies require time and repetition to assimilate the positive relationship overtures and to adjust internally. The transition can be observed as the behaviour changes. The art of observation and responsive care in services are key attributes to a practitioner's understanding and promotion of mental health in infants.

Stress

The hormone cortisol can have positive effects in the short term and negative for long-term periods if stress is prolonged. The circadian rhythm, as the 24-hour cycle of light and dark, regulates cortisol levels, but lifestyles can cause changes to these patterns. Many families do not adhere to the traditional pattern of sleep during darkness and activity during daylight hours. Parents express that they can spend prolonged sessions on internet activity during the night and struggle to cope with a waking baby in the early hours of sunrise. Long-term stress results in lengthy periods in which the body experiences high levels of cortisol which impacts adversely upon blood sugar, blood pressure, ability to sleep, and cognitive skill. Knowledge of the destructive properties of cortisol provides rationale to strategic planning and funding for intervention (National Scientific Council on the Developing Child, 2006). In addition, I feel that daily practice is greatly informed through understanding that excessive cortisol can stop neural connections occurring and create stress reactions which are barriers to learning and achievement of potential.

A high level of stress can also result in a stress response system being underactive. For example, a baby's lifestyle is profoundly disrupted if parenting skills are affected by toxic stress which the parent is unable to reduce. A baby experiences the negative impact of this stress albeit indirectly from the source that affects his parents. During these episodes, the baby's hippocampus, which is the area of the limbic system supporting memory and links to emotion and sensory learning, produces fewer cortisol receptors thus stress remains at a high level.

I have not heard the concept of learned helplessness applied to practice for many years, but the associated presentation is well known in a context of child protection and displayed within observations of infants and primary carers who have experienced abuse. The young child may appear to be placid and content to an inexperienced practitioner, or to a parent. The child may appear preoccupied with his proximal environment, particularly his own clothing or body. I observe children actively hiding from a perceived threat by covering their faces with hands or play items, moving under equipment, or shutting their eyes and dipping their heads downwards towards their chests.

I have frequently observed the presentation of some infants as being non-responsive and challenging for a practitioner to stimulate with learning opportunities. Primitive dissociative adaptations, and physical and cognitive freeze, are accompanied by physiological responses to prepare the body and mind for dealing with a forthcoming threat. The heart rate slows down, blood flows away from extremities, endogenous opioids reduce physical pain and may flood the mind with a sensation of calmness and psychological distancing from an attack. An infant who operates within a lifestyle of adversities learns to minimise the potential for stress by limiting human interaction despite the context of a nurturing nursery.

In the early stages of my career, the children who presented with these characteristics were termed *still children* which depicted their body language. During the 1980s, and 1990s, we observed and recorded this behaviour and sought to devise practical strategies that supported engagement. As practitioners, we did not have access to scientific knowledge or an opportunity to increase our understanding from research. Throughout a career, it is useful for practitioners to reflect upon previous practice, and historical memories, in order to enhance understanding. An increase in comprehension of the circumstances is valuable. Reflection is a key factor in gaining optimum value from work experiences and raising a practitioner's ability to link research, and practice, thus closing the implementation gap.

Box 1.2 Example from practice

A key worker called me into the baby room to observe our new nursery infant, Joy. I slipped quietly through the doorway which was festooned with brightly coloured ribbons and welcoming photographs, and I tucked myself into a corner of the warm playroom. I am well aware of the intrusive impact of an adult entering a playroom mid-session and disturbing the ambience between familiar practitioners and children. The key worker nodded towards Joy. I saw an infant of seven months with fine blond hair sitting steadily upon a patterned rug. The key worker called her name, and she gently rolled a soft red ball towards the little girl. A quiet bell emanated from the ball at each tumble. The ball had been constructed for play by babies or young infants, and the soft velvet material prevented this toy from reaching its destination upon the black-and-white checked rug.

Joy's body stiffened, her fists clenched, and she turned her head sharply to one side, averting gaze or potential interaction with this red intruder. Joy's body language depicted her uncertainty and indicated to staff that the little girl did not know how or where to seek help. She had not recognised the secure haven which the key worker offered. The practitioner touched the ball with two fingers to make it spin. The intention was not to invade the personal space of this fearful infant but to stimulate curiosity and potential learning from the proximal environment of a nursery playroom. The infant perceived an increase in threat level. Joy's head dipped forward, and she removed eye contact from her immediate surroundings.

Learned helplessness implies that the child has consciously acquired this behaviour; however, it is a demonstration of an instinctive protective reaction to external negative influences. The disconnection results in the child gaining some control over the threat by focusing inwards and minimising interpretation of the negative aspects. This strategy reduced the potential for emotional and physiological impact upon Joy's mind and body.

Social development

Social development of an infant is cultural and contextual. The first relationship and dyad in life before birth is the infant and his mother. By 26 weeks gestation, a foetus can react to the sound of his mother's voice, and hearing is known to be one of the first systems to develop.

At birth, babies demonstrate an intense interest in human faces and attempt to copy gestures. This important finding signifies learning through socialisation. Normative development indicates that socialisation progresses from a context of care routines at birth to a baby of 4 months seeking out stimulation of the wider environment beyond his care needs. Thereafter, an infant will make use of social referencing by adopting reactions and emotions of the primary carer as his world is extended.

The framework of reference that the baby uses to engage, to interact, and to understand the world evolves rapidly throughout the first year. The initial 12 months of life are regarded as one of the most sensitive periods for learning, and the baby should be supported to maintain physical and emotional health for genetic potential to be fulfilled. Babies learn at different rates, and the astute practitioner appreciates the importance of repetition and consolidation of knowledge to support understanding.

Care routines take place many times per day. These nurturing adult–child interactions provide perfect opportunities for a key worker to observe a baby's needs and interests and to support expansion of his inner working model. This internal framework is based upon experiential learning, and positive or negative emotions rapidly become associated with care patterns. Secure attachment is a key concept in services, and early years settings commonly operate with a key-worker system. This adult–child relationship is not an exclusive partnership, and an infant can create nurturing relationships with other staff and students in the age group in which he is based. Some early years services describe these room-worker relationships as positively extending the rationale of key worker, in a context of secure attachment and learning. During the pandemic, children in nurseries were cared for by a group of practitioners within a "care bubble" as opposed to designated key workers due to isolation periods impacting upon the service delivery.

Human beings continue to need secure attachment relationships throughout life to achieve and to support mental and emotional good health. Attachment is an adaptation to a set of circumstances. Insecure attachment is exhibited by an inability to self-regulate; therefore, the circumstances must change to promote agency and a sense of self. Balbernie (2013) explained that a value of poor should not be linked to attachment as the infant is simply demonstrating effective survival responses to adversities albeit he is not securely attached.

It is often the case that concerns about relationships are expressed as a child "not having secure attachment to an adult." Each infant has an inherent predisposition to seek out positive relationships with a primary carer from birth, but attachment requires a dyad in which an adult responds to a baby's emotional and physical needs and provides the optimum conditions for development. Strengthening of attachment occurs within every moment of interaction. The conditions nurture and respond to the baby's overtures for a supportive relationship.

The relationship with a primary carer is a template that informs future relational capacity, and it provides the infant with a medium in which he can learn to regulate emotions, behaviour, and actions. Lack of self-control, and a limited capacity to regulate, can create conditions of high vulnerability in childhood and potentially relational and mental-health issues in adulthood. Four aspects are identified by Balbernie (2013) as stress factors that can impact upon the infant–mother relationship.

1 Biological vulnerability of each infant.
2 Parental history of adversities and current parenting skills.
3 Interactional or parenting variables in each family.
4 Socio-demographic factors which may be influenced by a community.

Promotion, prevention, and intervention

In practice, I find that sources of stress are commonly described by parents as external factors in the form of environmental issues, for example, inadequate housing, poverty, and neighbourhood discrimination. Shonkoff and Fisher (2013) commented that daily financial stresses lead to families operating within crisis mode over long-term periods, which is associated with low self-regulatory skills. These authors stated that ability and capacity to plan and to receive delayed gratification is greatly reduced in a context of poverty.

Intervention should support development of parents and increase their capacity to manage the daily stresses. Two examples are the Head Start and High Scope programmes in the USA (Schweinhart, 2005). These innovative approaches to education and care were created in the 1960s in response to the needs of children living in poverty by targeting the potential for academic failure in the early school years. Findings indicated long-term benefits from preschool interventions for the children of families who existed in a context of daily poverty. Conclusions highlighted consistent patterns of cause and effect from preschool programmes of one or two years to achievement in adulthood. Achievement in this study of 123 participants included a reduction in episodes of criminality in relation to the norm, graduation from high-school education, and earnings in adulthood.

The initial programmes contributed to shaping parental interventions today, and consideration is given to location, staff skill, needs, and cultural characteristics of families, in addition to timing and duration of intervention. Some programmes commence in the prenatal period and focus upon a strengths-based model, for example, the Nurse–Family Partnership in the USA. In the UK, this programme is termed the Family Nurse Partnership (Family Nurse Partnership, 2011).

Toxic stress can affect the architecture of the brain, and this finding is significant to early intervention work and the necessity of supports by multi-agencies. Alleviation of these factors does not necessarily result in a reduction of toxic stress. Implicit memories which are based upon emotions can reproduce the stress reactions although the original source is minimised. Parents and grandparents will often recount historical instances of sexual abuse and exhibit emotions from a childlike perspective to service providers. It is challenging as a practitioner to respond with the optimum support as disclosures usually occur in unexpected circumstances. For example, within my work-place, the cloakroom area is a regular discussion venue for parents to exhibit help-seeking behaviours to professionals (Braun et al., 2006; Broadhurst, 2003; Whitters, 2015). Early years services are busy, active environments, and staff have to adhere to adult–child ratios at all times. Parents expect an immediate response to help-seeking cues. During this COVID-19 pandemic, parents cannot access service buildings, and other means of help-seeking communication have emerged, for example, by phone, text, and email.

Patterns of responses may evolve in relation to circumstances of toxic stress. These patterns result in physiological changes and associated repeated behaviours. Patterns which are created in the earliest years of childhood can persist throughout the lifespan and be activated by minor and major threats. Intervention by services, or positive role-modelling by an influential adult, can have a positive impact at any age. Changing the operational skills of an infant is best achieved through intervention with the extended family unit. Families require guidance in rethinking interpretation of their world, and subsequently the chemical reactions in the body will change and toxic stress reactions will reduce for an infant and his family.

Each registered workplace adheres to national care standards which give detailed expectation of the learning environments and skills required by practitioners to keep every child safe, healthy, achieving, nurtured, active, respected, responsible, and included. An example is the Scottish National Practice Model, termed Getting It Right for Every Child, and this document guides planning, practice, assessment, and child protection (Scottish Government, 2008, 2021). The model provides a context in which to implement the curricula: current Scottish curricula are Curriculum for Excellence (Scottish Government, 2004) and Pre-Birth to Three (Scottish Government, 2010). The four UK countries have similar curricula, and guidance is based upon the United Nations Rights of the Child (United Nations Convention on the Rights of the Child, 1989).

Curricular guidance is informed by research findings which additionally influence legislation. Early years practitioners have a responsibility to seek understanding from guidance and to apply knowledge within the context of their roles. Time to reflect is a necessary condition of professional develop-ment. Many care and education settings use "clean-down" time for collegiate discussion. Sorting and sterilising equipment and preparing a learning envir-onment provide repetitive but therapeutic activities for an early years team. This type of group professional reflection has great value due to the local context and relevance to timely discussion of a concern or celebration of a family's progress.

The study by Thompson et al. (2019) identified an increase in cortisol of a participant group of children throughout the period of a day spent in early years care. Findings indicated an increase in activation and overtaxing of the stress response systems. The control group of children who remained at home did not demonstrate an increase in this stress hormone. The research team described three common sources of adversity in families: low socio-economic status, mental-health issues relating to the mother, and child abuse. The study did not portray the day-care environment as directly contributing to stress but implied that the environment did not alleviate the stress experienced by the children. This finding is informative for early years services. Practitioners cannot change the lifestyles of families, but a key responsibility is supporting the child's resilience and changing the local environment to reduce any negative impacts upon learning and development.

Three brain systems which are susceptible to toxic stress are emotional regulation, memory, and executive functioning. Constant states of agitation can also impact negatively upon the immune system. In 2018, the American Heart Association advised that emphasis should be given to interventions that reduce exposure to adversity in childhood as a preventative measure to chronic inflammation throughout adulthood. Short-term adaptations to stress have been linked to long-term consequences of adversity, for example, maladaptive behaviour, an acceleration of the ageing process, chronic illness in adulthood, and a shortened lifespan (National Scientific Council on the Developing Child, 2020).

It is known that relationships and environment affect the emotional development of young children. A high level of cortisol during waking hours has been linked to negative emotions of infants, alongside maternal depression. Infants who exhibit higher than average cortisol levels demonstrate characteristics which can also be observed in depressed adults. Examples cited by Luby and Whalen (2019) included a distinct lack of mood change from negative to positive in a context of environmental stimulation, inconsistent sleep patterns, and alteration to daily appetite.

Luby and Whalen (2019) conducted research on depression in early childhood, and these authors described infants as young as 2 months old displaying negative emotions, which included sadness. At 6 months of age, infants were demonstrating sad and joyful expressions. These reactions corresponded to events in the study which were designed to create negative or positive emotion. Behaviour associated with depression in infants includes withdrawal from proximal stimulation in the environment, apathy, and failure to thrive. Improving the infant's relationship with a primary carer is regarded as a key aspect of intervention.

In the earliest years of life, the infant's emotional arousal is regulated by a responsive parent or practitioner. Tronick and Beeghly (2011) described how infants create a bio-psychosocial state of consciousness by use of non-verbal meaning. Making meaning is an iterative, lifelong process that is individual to each infant and influenced by multiple internal and external drivers. The infant's interpretation of his world is demonstrated by movement, actions, and emotions. The adult–child dyad supports the infant to increase his comprehension of the proximal world by reference to other beings and to himself. Emotional regulation, effective communication skills, expression of emotions, social competence, and the capacity to explore an environment are indicators of good mental health.

However, if a carer's capacity to support an infant is compromised, then the infant may struggle to develop and to maintain emotional homeostasis as termed by Thompson (1991). Jennings et al. (2008) studied 134 infants to explore potential links between development of self-regulation, comprehension of the autobiographical self, and maternal sensitivity to an infant's needs and emotions. Findings had revealed that an infant's ability to use his vision, and his eye contact to gain attention can be contributory factors to predicting development of self-regulation skills. A mother's warmth towards her child prompted motivation to learn, and children in this study appeared to adopt and to strive towards their mothers' goals. The conclusion indicated that maternal depression could affect the infant's capacity to gain self-regulation. Experiences that focused upon internal and external influences upon the child were recommended.

Experiences are influenced greatly by the culture and beliefs of each family, and particularly the interpretation of the world which is given to the infant by a primary carer, usually his mother (Rosenblum et al. 2019). Thompson (1991) described regulation as intrinsic and extrinsic processes that influence emotional reactions. Examples of intrinsic processes are language, cognitive skills, and the development of a sense of self. Extrinsic processes include parental and key-worker strategies and experiences that provide opportunities for the management of emotions and, ultimately, development of self-regulation.

Emotional experiences are affected by socialisation, and meanings are acquired that are pertinent to the individual and family. Over time, the young child's ability to regulate his emotions provides a foundation for his comprehension of others. For example, the child's expectations of emotional reactions are associated with social functioning in different contexts, and the personalities of his primary carer, extended family carers, and other significant adults. Thompson (1991) comments that social competence, cognitive functioning, and academic achievement are influenced by these stages of emotional development.

This increase in knowledge and understanding is embedded within the infant's behavioural processes, and emotions can quickly be associated with the infant's reaction to extrinsic influences from the environment. The management of emotion evolves from the nervous system (Thompson, 1991), which is immature at birth, therefore dependent on extrinsic influences to support development and capacity. There are two significant stages in inhibitory control at approximately 4 months and 10 months of age. Activation of emotional reactions can be positive and negative for an infant. For example, heightened emotions can stimulate and invigorate the young child by focusing his attention and facilitating learning. Emotions can support an infant to respond rapidly to changes in self or environment and to maintain a high level of engagement and interaction. Additionally, positive emotions prompt the use of memory and creation of relationships which can complement and capitalise upon learning opportunities. Alternatively, negative emotional reaction can create a barrier to knowledge acquisition if an infant is focused upon coping with an adversity and maintaining his perceived or actual safety.

Rosenblum et al. (2019) applied two theoretical perspectives to the under-standing of human emotions: the structuralist and fundamentalist approaches. Structuralists associate behaviour and timescales with emotions. Fundamentalists emphasise the relational aspects of emotions by linking to specific stimuli and preparing the infant for action. Risk and protective factors can hinder or enhance development, and infants encounter multiple potentially adverse factors throughout their earliest years. Biological factors are often regarded as the most obvious source of negative influence, for example, prematurity, accompanying low birth weight, and additional learning needs.

Research by Schechter et al. (2019) indicated that an infant's capacity to recall events is increasingly evident throughout the first year of life, although the ability to comprehend experiences emerges over time alongside language and communication skills. Adversity which is chronic or a single event which has an extreme impact upon the infant may result in dissociation, and affect recall and neurobiology of the brain.

The Centre on the Social and Emotional Foundations for Early Learning (2007) identified areas of adversity and strengths in families which may be adapted for use within assessment processes. These are family make-up, parenting skills, extended family influences, stress and responses by a family, infant's personality and particular strengths, family and community culture, and, finally, communication and emotional expression.

Larrieu et al. (2019) described dimensions of the caregiving environment and the infant's characteristics as providing a framework for determining intervention which is based upon the strengths of each family. The caregiving environment encompasses the primary carer's ability to conduct problem-solving, conflict resolution, understand role and responsibilities, communicate instrumentally, and respond to emotions. Additionally, to demonstrate emotional investment, support behavioural regulation and coordination, and maintain sibling harmony. Infant characteristics that affect implementation of an intervention include temperament, sensory awareness, physical and mental health, learning style, and developmental status (Zero to Three, 2016). Intentional communication by an infant is also an important factor in intervention. In the early stages of childhood, communication is characterised by three functions: behaviour regulation, joint attention, and social interaction (Saletta & Windsor, 2019). These areas are described in later chapters of this book.

The research of Beebe et al. (2012) focused upon the use of a dyadic system to support positive development of a secure attachment relationship and internal working model in an infant. This system incorporates joint coordination as expressed by these authors. Each person in the dyad coordinates his behaviour with the other. Another term which is used in practice is the dance of reciprocity. Daily care routines, in addition to exploration of an environment, provide contexts for intrapersonal and interpersonal rhythms to evolve. Routines present multiple opportunities for emotional patterns to be created, or changed, as the infant's comprehension of his sense of self matures.

Findings from the aforementioned research indicated that the infant learns by his own experience and the experience of the other person in this dyadic system; thus, the participants are interdependent on one another.

Beebe et al. (2012) promote three principles to interactions within the dyadic system of adult and infant: ongoing regulations, disruption and repair, and heightened affective moments. As the interaction progresses, each participant recreates a psychophysiological state in the sense of self which is similar to that of his partner in the dyad. If a mother is unable to achieve this level of comprehension of the infant's state, then her empathy towards her child is affected adversely (Beebe et al. 2012).

Responses to infant mental health encompass promotion, prevention, and intervention to minimise the impact of negative influences in the earliest stages of life (Centre on the Social and Emotional Foundations for Early Learning, 2007). A strategic and operational approach is to extend the infant's experiences, environmental and relational, and to actively support his mental health. Zeanah et al. (2005) identify three principles of infant mental health.

1   Consistent relationships as building blocks of social and emotional development.
2   Use of a continuum of services which can be matched to family needs and preferences.
3   Finally, training and supervision of the practitioner workforce.

Intervention aims to activate or to increase the infant's capacity and to achieve positive outcomes by using a strengths-based approach. The common target areas for intervention are described below.

- The parent–child, practitioner–child, and practitioner–parent relationships.
- A positive environmental context for learning that supports social and emotional well-being and associated behaviours.
- Continuous professional development of the workforce, which promotes an increase in knowledge, understanding, reflection, and practical expertise in infant mental health.

Assessment of the primary carer to infant relationship is essential to determine responsive intervention for each dyad. Consideration must also be given to nurturing potential in a context of supportive practitioner–infant and practitioner–parent relationships. The practitioner–parent relationship is a key feature in family services which can effectively link the micro-systems of home and playroom. Partnership skills with child and parent develop over time through experiential learning. Professional characteristics in the context of infant mental health are the ability to listen and to consider, to reflect on positive and negative influences upon each infant and self, to increase knowledge, and significantly to gain deeper understanding.

References

Association of Infant Mental Health, UK. (2021). The infant mental health competency framework. https://aimh.uk/the-uk-imh-competency-framework.

Balbernie, R. (2013). The importance of secure attachment for infant mental health. *Journal of Health Visiting*, 1(*4*), 210–217.

Beebe, B., Lachmann, F., Markese, S., & Bahrick, L. (2012). On the origins of disorganised attachment and internal working models: Paper 1, a dyadic systems approach. *Psychoanalytic Dialogues: The International Journal of Relational Perspectives*, 22(*2*), 253–272.

Berens, A. E., & Nelson, C. A. (2019). Neurobiology of foetal and infant development. In C. H. Zeanah (Ed.), *Handbook of infant mental health*, 4th edition (pp. 41–62). New York: The Guilford Press.

Bowlby, J. (1979). *The making and breaking of affectional bonds.* Abingdon and New York: Routledge.

Braun, D., Davis, H., & Mansfield, P. (2006). *How helping works: Towards a shared model of process.* London: The Centre for Parent and Child Support.

Broadhurst, K. (2003). Engaging parents and carers with family support services: What can be learned from research on help-seeking? *Journal of Child and Family Social Work*, 8(*4*), 341–350.

Bronfenbrenner, U. (1979). *The ecology of human development*, 2nd edition. Cambridge, MA: Harvard University Press.

Bronfenbrenner, U. (2005). *Making human beings human: Biological perspectives on human development.* Thousand Oaks, CA: Sage Publications.

Bronfenbrenner, U. & Morris, P. A. (2006). The bioecological model of human development. In W. Damon & R. M. Lerner (Eds.), *Handbook of child psychology*, vol. I (pp. 796–798, 800, 810–815). Hoboken, NJ: Wiley & Sons.

Cassidy, J., & Mohr, J. J. (2001). Unsolvable fear, trauma, and psychopathology: Theory, research and clinical considerations related to disorganized attachment across the life span. *Clinical Psychology: Science and Practice*, 8(*3*), 275–298.

Centre for Excellence and Outcomes in Children and Young People's Services (C4EO) (2010). *Grasping the nettle: Early intervention for children, families and communities* (pp. 5, 49–50). London: Local Government Management Board.

Centre on the Social and Emotional Foundations for Early Learning (2007). *Infant mental health and early care and education providers.* https://www.csefel.vanderbilt.edu/documents/rs_infant_mental_health.pdf.

Dismukes, A. R., Shirtcliff, E. A., & Drury, S. S. (2019). Genetic and epigenetic processes in infant mental health. In C. H. Zeanah (Ed.), *Handbook of infant mental health*, 4th edition (pp. 63–80). New York: The Guilford Press.

Family Nurse Partnership (2011). The evaluation of the family nurse partnership programme in Scotland: Phase 1 report – intake and early pregnancy. https://www.gov.scot/publications/evaluation-family-nurse-partnership-programme-scotland-phase-1-report-intake-early-pregnancy/.

Fogel, A. (1982). Social play, positive affect, and coping skills in the first 6 months of life. *Early Childhood Special Education*, 2(*3*), 53–65.

Gerhardt, S. (2004). *Why love matters: How affection shapes a baby's brain.* Hove: Routledge.

Jennings, K. D., Sandberg, I., Kelley, S. A., Valdes, L., Yaggi, K., Abrew, A., & Macey-Kalcevic, M. (2008). Understanding of self and maternal warmth predict later self-regulation in toddlers. *International Journal of Behavioural Development*, 32(2), 108–118.

Laevers, F. (1994). *The project experiential education: Concepts and experiences at level of context, process, and outcome.* Leuven: Leuven University.

Larrieu, J. A., Middleton, M. A., Kelley, A. C., & Zeanah, C. H. (2019). Assessing the relational context of infants and young children. In C. H. Zeanah (Ed.), *Handbook of infant mental health*, 4th edition (pp. 279–295). New York: The Guilford Press.

Luby, J. L., & Whalen, D. (2019). Depression in early childhood. In C. H. Zeanah (Ed.), *Handbook of infant mental health*, 4th edition (pp. 426–437). New York: The Guilford Press.

National Scientific Council on the Developing Child. (2006). Early exposure to toxic substances damages brain architecture. Working paper no. 4. https://developingchild.harvard.edu/resources/early-exposure-to-toxic-substances-damages-brain-architecture.

National Scientific Council on the Developing Child. (2020). Connecting the brain to the rest of the body: Early childhood development and lifelong health are deeply intertwined. Working paper number 15. http://developingchild.harvard.edu/wp-con tent/uploads/2020/06/wp15_health_FINAL_061520.pdf.

NHS Education for Scotland. (2019). *Perinatal mental health curricular framework: A framework for maternal and infant mental health.* https://learn.nes.nhs.scot/10383/perinatal-and-infant-mental-health/perinatal-mental-health-curricular-framework-a-framework-for-maternal-and-infant-mental-health.

Rosenblum, K. L., Dayton, C. J., & Muzik, M. (2019). Infant social and emotional development, emerging competence in a relational context. In C. H. Zeanah (Ed.), *Handbook of infant mental health*, 4th edition (pp. 95–119). New York: The Guilford Press.

Saletta, M. & Windsor, J. (2019). Communication disorders in infants and children. In C. H. Zeanah (Ed.), *Handbook of infant mental health*, 4th edition (pp. 345–357). New York: The Guilford Press.

Schechter, D. S., Wilheim, E., Suardi, F., & Serpa, S. R. (2019). The effects of violent experiences on infants and young children. In C. H. Zeanah (Ed.), *Handbook of infant mental health*, 4th edition (pp. 219–238). New York: The Guilford Press.

Schweinhart, L. J. (2005). The High/Scope Perry preschool study through age 40 summary, conclusions, and frequently asked questions. https://image.highscope.org/wp-content/uploads/2018/11/16053615/perry-preschool-summary-40.

Scottish Government. (2004). *A curriculum for excellence.* Edinburgh: Scottish Government.

Scottish Government. (2008). *A guide to getting it right for every child.* Edinburgh: Scottish Government.

Scottish Government. (2010). *Pre-birth to three: Positive outcomes for Scotland's children and families.* Edinburgh: Scottish Government.

Scottish Government. (2019). *Engaging parents and families.* Edinburgh: Scottish Government.

Scottish Government. (2021). *National guidance for child protection 2021.* Edinburgh: Scottish Government.

Shonkoff, J. P., & Fisher, P. A. (2013). Re-thinking evidence-based practice and two-generation programmes to create the future of early childhood practice. *Developmental psychology*, 25, 1635–1653.

Shonkoff, J. P., Slopen, N., & Williams, D. R. (2021). Early childhood adversity, toxic stress, and the impacts of racism on the foundations of health. *Annual Review of Public Health*, 42, 115–134.

Slade, A., & Sadler, L. S. (2019). Pregnancy and infant mental health. In C. H. Zeanah (Ed.), *Handbook of infant mental health*, 4th edition (pp. 25–40). New York: The Guilford Press.

Sloan, H., & Donnelly, R. (2021). From "bumps to bundles": Perinatal mental health in NHS greater Glasgow and Clyde. https://www.academia.edu/6198962/From_Bumps_to_Bundles_Perinatal_Mental_Health_in_NHS_Greater_Glasgow_and_Clyde_Contents.

Stern, D. N. (1985). *The interpersonal world of the infant*. London: H. Karnac.

Thompson, R. A. (1991). Emotional regulation and emotional development. *Educational Psychology Review*, 3(*4*), 269–307.

Thompson, S. F., Kiff, C. J., & McLaughlin, K. A. (2019). The neurobiology of stress and adversity in infancy. In C. H. Zeanah (Ed.), *Handbook of infant mental health*, 4th edition (pp. 81–94). New York: The Guilford Press.

Trevarthan, C., and Aitken, K. J. (2001). Infant intersubjectivity: research, theory, and clinical applications. *Journal of Child Psychology and Psychiatry*, 42(*1*), 3–48.

Tronick, E., & Beeghly, M. (2011). Infants' meaning-making and the development of mental health problems. *American Psychology*, 66(*2*), 107–109.

United Nations Convention on the Rights of the Child (1989). *United Nations convention on the rights of the child*. Geneva: United Nations.

Weatherston, D. (2000). The infant mental health specialist. *Zero to Three: National Centre for Infants, Toddlers, and Families*.

Whitters, H. G. (2015). Perceptions of the influences upon the parent-professional relationship in a context of early intervention and child protection. Ph.D. thesis, University of Strathclyde.

World Association for Infant Mental Health. (2000). Mission statement overview. https://waimh.org/general/custom.asp?page=about_waimh.

Zeanah, C. H., Carter, A. S., Cohen, J., Egger, H., Gleason, M. M., Keren, M., Lieberman, A., Mulrooney, K., & Oser, C. (2016). Diagnostic classification of mental health and developmental disorders of infancy and early childhood DC:0–5. *Infant Mental Health Journal*, 37(*5*), 471–475.

Zeanah, C. H., & Zeanah, P. D. (2019). Infant mental health: The clinical science of experience. In C. H. Zeanah (Ed.), *Handbook of infant mental health*, 4th edition (pp. 5–24). New York: The Guilford Press.

Zeanah, P. D., Stafford, B. S., Nagle, G. A., & Rice, T. (2005). *Addressing social-emotional development and infant mental health in early childhood systems*,12. Los Angeles, CA: National Center for Infant and Early Childhood Health Policy.

2 Relationships, involvement, and well-being

Chapter 2 focuses upon the infant's relationships and the impact upon well-being and involvement with a learning environment. The chapter describes the infant's demonstration of attachment behaviours from birth (Howe, 2005). Separation protest and proximity-seeking are key behavioural systems that are expressed in the early years. Discussion is presented of the bio-social homeostatic regulatory system and includes reciprocal adult attachment behaviour (Fonagy, 1999). Babies are unable to regulate their emotional reactions at birth; however, the dyadic system develops over time, and it creates an essential baseline of knowledge and understanding for the developing infant (Fukkink, 2021).

Transgenerational transmission of deprivation is described alongside intervention that can support families to change and to develop in a context of daily living. Three significant aspects of change to the inner working models of primary carers that support infant mental health are highlighted: behavioural, cognitive, and social. Attunement, reciprocity, marked mirroring, containment, and reflective functioning are described as contributing to the ability and capacity of an infant to adapt to different environments and relationships. The Circle of Security (Cooper et al., 2016) and the Solihull Approach (Douglas & Rheeston, 2009) are presented as interventions that support development of a secure interdependent family unit.

Relationships

Creation of a relationship with another fellow being is an inherent need of every infant, and a secure attachment relationship is the foundation for a healthy and fulfilling life. Infants demonstrate attachment behaviours from birth, for example, seeking close physical contact, holding tightly onto an adult, and showing preference for familiar human faces and voices with particular emphasis on eye contact with a mother. Separation protest and proximity-seeking are key behavioural systems that are expressed in the early years. Fonagy (1999) found that reciprocal adult attachment behaviour responds to and encourages the relationship overtures of an infant. Interactions lead to the infant experiencing security on a physical and emotional level. Babies are

DOI: 10.4324/9781003358107-2

unable to regulate their emotional reactions at birth; however, the dyadic system develops over time, and it creates an essential baseline of knowledge and understanding for the developing infant. In the early stages, regulation is based upon the infant's expectations and role-modelling from the primary carer's behaviour. Fonagy (1999) applied the term "bio-social homeostatic regulatory system" to these processes.

Bonding is presented as the emotional relationship from adult to child, and *attachment* is the child's emotional bond with the parent or a primary care-giver (Association of Infant Mental Health, UK, 2021).

These terms are often used interchangeably by carers. A caregiver can be closely associated with a proximal environment, for example, a parent within the home or a key worker in a nursery. During teaching sessions on relationship processes to parents, and practitioners, I feel that it is important to communicate that the infant does not have responsibility for creating a secure attachment relationship with an adult. Attachment requires a dyad, and the adult must present appropriate conditions and a responsive relationship in order for the child's attachment cues to be recognised and to support his status of emotional well-being and safety.

The Royal College of Midwives (2020) present common terms relating to infant mental health: "attunement", "reciprocity", "marked mirroring", "containment", "reflective functioning". These terms can be applied to describe actions that promote a positive attachment relationship and bonding between adult and infant.

- **Attunement**: the sharing of emotions between parent and infant as a response to an external influence, the baby's internal influences, or a positive emotional reaction to the parent–child relationship itself. A baby's internal influence is often detected by demonstration of physiological changes. After feeding, a baby may burp excess wind, and the parent celebrates this achievement with a positive emotion which the baby will thereafter associate with his internal sensation.
- **Reciprocity**: a parent described reciprocity to me as the "back and forward game". This descriptor accurately implies the turn-taking and creative aspect of reciprocity. The parent observes the baby's cues and quickly gives a response that meets the needs and interests as expressed by a cue. The baby initially copies the carer's body language and develops the interaction by use of his personality and changing needs at a point of time. Reciprocity incurs attunement, a feeling of great satisfaction by parent and infant, and entails a rich source of learning.
- **Marked mirroring**: a parent represents the infant's emotion by copying his expression which is often prompted by internal positive or negative influences and by supporting emotional containment. The baby may feel contented after a feed and change or express anxiety as a response to hunger and discomfort. A parent interprets his emotion by reference to knowledge of the baby's usual reactions to common circumstances.

Repetitive care processes each day provide a parent or practitioner with numerous opportunities to determine the baby's personality, specific characteristics, and reactions to his world.

- **Containment**: practitioners often receive training on the use of containment and strategies to support emotional expressions by parent and child. Adults can learn to contain a baby's emotions and to support his regulation without adopting the emotions.
- **Reflective functioning**: this is an essential aspect of childcare and education, and a parenting role. An adult caregiver considers the infant's individual needs, wants, and interests and presents a sensitive response in order to assuage these needs.

In 1954, Abraham Maslow described the hierarchy of needs in ascending order as physiological needs, safety and security, love and belonging, self-esteem, and self-actualisation (Maslow, 2000). Maslow determined that needs which were met created a foundation for further needs to be realised, and to be responded to by primary carers and community.

Bonding

Research indicates a link between maternal oxytocin levels and bonding between mother and foetus, and mother and infant (Royal College of Midwives, 2020). Low levels are associated with higher incidence of postnatal depression. During a Caesarean section there is no oxytocin released during the process. There is a delay of 48 hours before oxytocin is detected after this assisted birth (Levine et al., 2007). However, skin-to-skin contact between a newborn infant and mother has been found conducive to prompt oxytocin release at birth (UNICEF, 2021). In many countries, a newborn will be placed upon his mother's chest at birth to encourage the attachment processes and a bond which will last a lifetime.

The parent–child dyad supports the newborn to regulate his emotional reaction to external influences in the context of responses to objects, people, environmental conditions, and his changing internal physiological state. Acquiring and maintaining a status of emotional and physical security forms the rationale of the human attachment system, and seeking to achieve this goal is a motivational force upon the infant's behaviour. Adequate resources for development are required in the form of a variety of experiences, consistent relationships, and time for reflection that supports the infant to absorb and assimilate knowledge within his inner working model. His reactions, actions, and behaviour increase in complexity and intent over time. As the bio-social homeostatic regulatory system evolves, then the infant's ability and capacity to demonstrate resilience to adversity increases, and negative influences have less impact upon development.

Attachment is described in theory (Bowlby, 1979) as a bio-behavioural mechanism which is demonstrated as a response to anxiety and founded upon an outcome of survival. Observation of practice indicates that confirmation and consolidation of the attachment relationship occurs during an infant's exploration of his environment. The attachment system is not activated but maintained and strengthened during this time within adult–child reciprocal interactions. The dyadic regulation of affect encompasses the primary carer and infant working in partnership to achieve stability of the child's emotional states. Attachment is based upon needs and strategies associated with survival, in addition to supporting up-regulation and down-regulation of emotions encountered during learning.

Howe (2005) presents the child's organisation of attachment behaviours. Over time, the child's inner working model acquires representations of himself within a proximal environment, his interpretation of other people, and expectations of a relationship based upon his personal perspective and actions of others. This base of knowledge leads to the child's *use* of attachment behaviours to increase the responses from primary carers to his need for availability, and responsivity. His behaviour is communication about his needs and often indicates how an attachment figure can respond to these needs at a point of time. For example, an infant who desires physical reassurance will cry, give eye contact to a primary carer, and raise both arms to indicate that he wants to be lifted. If the adult lifts the child, then he will move his head towards her body and hold onto her clothing with both hands. This reinforces the message to the child that his communication methods are effective, and it provides the carer with the knowledge and practical skill that responds effectively to the particular attachment behaviour of this infant. The carer and child adapt their behaviour and create a goal-corrected partnership as termed by Howe (2005).

Fonagy (1999) expressed that activation of the attachment system is dependent on the child's interpretation of his world and resultant status of security, or insecurity. However, a child's understanding of environmental influences can also be led by the reaction of his parent or carer. The primary carer's reaction is based upon an adult inner working model which in itself was influenced by childhood experiences, positive and negative. Research indicates that children who are insecurely attached often have parents with a similar attachment status, which Fonagy termed the transgenerational transmission of deprivation.

Attachment behaviour includes over-regulation, in which the child is preoccupied with seeking care responses, or under-regulation, in which the child may avoid potential stress. A disorganised care environment does not support the child to identify or to use patterns of seeking and gaining secure attachment responses. Children who have experienced chaotic and inconsistent caregiving may perceive adults as a source of fear *and* reassurance. Anxiety is experienced by an infant as internal physiological changes in response to the behaviour of one specific adult, family members within a household, or strangers in a community (Fonagy, 1999). Behavioural patterns can exist in the context of chaotic households, but the complexity of identifying, and using, these patterns to support mental stability is beyond the developmental capability of most infants.

Circle of Security

Acquiring the skill of reflective functioning is significant to the development of secure attachment capacity in parents whose relationships are influenced by their own childhood adversities. Fonagy (1999) presents potential for change in a parent's behaviour if opportunities and interventions can specifically support the development of this skill. In turn, a parent's increase in reflective functioning instigates reflection in the child, and this intersubjective process contributes to the development of their secure attachment relationship. The Circle of Security (Cooper et al., 2016) and the Solihull Approach (Douglas & Rheeston, 2009) are used within my workplace to train practitioners and parents in the rationale and behaviour associated with reflective functioning between adult and child. The primary carer, as an attachment figure, provides two main functions:

1   A safe haven from potential threat. Threat may relate to new and unpre-
    dictable environments or a young child's inability to differentiate between
    safety and danger. This haven is communicated to the child by the adult's
    body language, availability, and reassurance through role-modelling from
    the perspective of an adult's interpretation of the potential danger. In
    addition, attuning to the child's changing emotions and behaviour as his
    knowledge and understanding increases confirms the status of an envir-
    onment being safe for exploration. A safe haven refers to the attachment
    figure and not the environmental setting, although a primary carer can
    present a positive interpretation of an environment to the child by her
    behaviour and attitude.

2   A secure base results in the attachment system being deactivated as the
    child recognises conditions which are conducive to exploration, discovery,
    and learning about his proximal and distal world. In practice, the child
    does continue to refer to his attachment figure during these forays and to
    share his delight in discovery through eye contact and body language.
    Infants will often return to the attachment figure every few moments to
    gain reassurance. I ask parents to imagine a string of elastic thread con-
    joining adult and infant. It can be stretched over time, but the connection
    remains constant. If an adult responds consistently to a child's relational
    overtures, usually by the use of gesture or verbal interaction, then the
    attachment relationship will be consolidated.

Secure and insecure are usually the attachment classifications given to parents as a baseline for understanding their role and infant's behaviours. These
two descriptors represent the child's emotional well-being in a context of the
parent–child relationship. Secure, ambivalent, avoidant, and chaotic are

further descriptors that support practitioners to recognise and interpret these behaviours. A child can have different categories of relationships with adults and siblings since attachment is a reciprocal phenomenon that depends on a carer's responses to the child's initiations.

Relationship dyad

Difficulties in forming positive relationships do not just affect the individual but impact upon the relationship dyad, and the behaviour of one partner may be detrimental to the other. The establishment of secure attachment with a key worker in a service can provide a change in understanding and expectations of a relationship with a *parent* for an insecurely attached infant. However, if the parent is unable to change his or her attachment responses and to provide a safe haven and secure base, then the infant will remain insecurely attached to his mother or father. Sroufe et al. (2000) linked physical abuse, lack of emotional care, and empathy to conduct and anxiety issues in a child. This research suggested that formation of a positive relationship with an adult who is not a primary carer, for example, a grandparent or a professional, can mitigate the negative effects of a parent–child relationship.

Doyle (2001) conducted a small significant study twenty years ago that highlighted the influence of comfort objects in a context of attachment and security. The participant group was composed of 14 adult survivors of childhood emotional abuse. Findings indicated that the parents of some of the participants had experienced difficulties in demonstrating love but had allowed children to create positive relationships with others. These children had gained nurture from comfort toys, pet animals, or personal artefacts. Participants in this study had identified contact with pets as a key source of impactful relationships in childhood.

The aforementioned study cites play-therapy sessions as contributing to an accumulation of positive experiences for a child, although these sessions do not directly impact on changing parental behaviour (Doyle, 2001). It is known that interventions based upon play-therapy principles can have a major impact upon a child's resilience to adversity, and his ability and capacity to minimise the negative effects upon his sense of self can increase. Previous studies have shown that parents may attempt to block opportunities for a child to form relationships with other significant people, and the research by Farmer and Owen (1995) indicated that parents may actively sabotage these relationships. The authors present an example of a child's relationship with a play therapist.

Doyle (2001) concluded that social support does not have to be intense or even long-lasting in order to gain a long-term effect on a child's security and positive sense of self. One or more positive relationships can be supplemented by the use of comfort objects or pets. Due to restrictions imposed by the current COVID-19 pandemic, to minimise potential for virus transfer, children cannot bring personal objects into a service from home. However, the key-worker relationship is formed in the early moments of induction, and this strategy has supported creation of a secure attachment between practitioner and child. Forming patterns of behaviour during transitions are significant representations of a safe haven that are retained by each child integrating into a service. Implicit memories are formed that can reconfigure the inner working model and promote a positive blueprint of relationships to the young child. Transition from home to nursery can be supported by the use of a nursery toy in place of a home toy as representative of a safe haven. The final finding from this research indicated that the cumulative effect of multiple positive experiences is a key aspect to healthy social and emotional development within the context of adversities.

Separation anxiety

Sroufe et al. (2000) linked challenging relationships to a disorder in the category of psychopathology. *Separation anxiety* is one illustration of a relationship problem. This condition is one of the effects of the COVID-19 pandemic which is currently being exhibited in services. Infants are referred for placement who have not experienced life outside the home environment due to lockdown conditions throughout the country. Many infants have adopted the high level of anxiety and stress that is being experienced and exhibited by their parents on a daily basis. The continuation of COVID-19 procedures and regulations has meant that parents are unable to enter a service.

This set of circumstances may appear detrimental to the formation of a key-worker–infant relationship in a context of separation anxiety. In reality, many anecdotal reports from services indicate that families can cope with the home-to-nursery transition more effectively than pre-COVID. Infants and parents appear to be compartmentalising their relationships to specific contexts and minimising transition anxiety. Due to COVID conditions, the transition is focused upon two people: the parent and key worker representing a relational person-to-person transition bridge. Each attachment figure is located within a specific environment: the parent is outside a service that represents the home environment; and the key worker is inside a service. Previously a parent would create a person–environmental transition bridge between home and nursery by entering a service with the child. I feel that key workers have benefited from these necessary health and safety conditions by focusing with greater intent, purpose, and understanding on the creation of a secure attachment relationship with an infant. The practitioner has gained an increase in self-worth and value of his relationship with key children.

Self-regulation

The ability and capacity to adapt one's behaviour and actions to different environments, and relationships with others, are unique to human beings (Tomasello, 1999). These skills encompass comprehension of other people as being intentional mental agents which is gained within a specific species and a social group culture. In the early stages of infancy, and throughout childhood, a baby relies on sensitive responding from a primary carer to co-regulate his emotions. As the months progress over the first year of life, the infant develops purpose in his actions and begins to direct his caregiver. The infant is influenced at the behavioural and physiological level, and he gains an elementary ability and capacity to make decisions in relation to his felt needs. The self-regulation processes evolve throughout a lifespan from a foundation that is created during infancy.

By the end of the first year, an infant has the capacity to use learning skills in the form of gaze, absorption of information, followed by social referencing, and imitation. Tomasello (1999) refers to triadic interactions at this stage of development in which the infant's focus is extended from self to a primary carer, and their shared interest in the proximal environment. This research study found that 12-month-old infants copied intentional actions of a primary carer which were used for a specific purpose, and the infants ignored accidental actions by the adult. Furthermore, findings indicated that infants could apply the intentional actions to multiple circumstances, which increased their skill sets and extended cultural learning.

The infant begins to understand his ability to direct an adult's attention to his chosen object or area of exploration by the use of direct gesture or subtle body language. In services, the practitioners will use observations and information-sharing with parents to acquire intimate knowledge of an infant's personality, interests at a point in time, and communication strategies. The child's perception of his own mental state depends on ability and capacity to notice his caregiver's representation of their shared world and to create a foundation of knowledge and understanding for personal use. Imaginative or pretend play between an adult and child provides multiple opportunities for the developing infant to be guided towards an understanding of reality in his external world through his internal representation of these experiences. The parent's involvement with the child's internal world, in a context of imaginative play, supports development of an understanding of self as an intentional mental agent. Over time, the child can appreciate that his imaginative world does not need to replicate his external experiences. Imagination and creativity lead to the child gaining mastery, control, and increase in self-esteem by exploring and consolidating his ideas and understanding.

During the teleological period, in the development of self, the child interprets behaviour of others within a context of visible outcomes, as opposed to non-concrete beliefs. The infant may experience anxiety, or satisfaction, with reference to his internal physiological changes and interpretation of the external environment. The infant's body and mind are in a state of arousal. His experience includes representation of the world by his primary carer, usually the mother, foster carer, or key worker in the earliest days and months. The infant's behaviour is initially a representation of his internal experiences and reactions. Patterns can rapidly evolve, and persist, particularly if the infant is exposed to situations that induce chronic anxiety.

Mirroring

Mirroring is a key learning medium at this early stage of development, and infants will copy, and assimilate, a parent's interpretation and emotional reaction to circumstances or events. A mother's interpretative signals will incorporate her personal comprehension allied with historical life influences and encompass her parenting goals and attempts to guide her infant. Bowlby (1979) applied the term of "inner working model", which is a framework of reference for the operational skills and executive functioning of human beings, based upon prior experiences and interpretations of the world. The inner working model is influenced by a cultural context that reflects family or community attitudes, in addition to parental values and beliefs that support decision-making.

Marked mirroring, as described previously, is a term that is applied to this context. A primary carer may briefly reflect her infant's emotion then present a representation that supports containment of his negative emotions. The adult is momentarily experiencing the infant's negative emotion and activating his or her own regulation skills to react resiliently. This experiential learning scenario can occur many times within a daily lifestyle at home or within services. Fonagy (1999) describes this period as supportive of symbol formation. The infant is given information to extend his understanding of internal self and external representation in this intersubjective process with a primary carer. Comprehension matures over time, and meaning gains complexity as multiple experiences are presented to the infant. The caregiver's response to the child is assimilated with a representation of his physical, emotional, and mental state. This knowledge is stored within the infant's inner working model and will be refined, consolidated, or reconfigured over time.

Sensitive responding

Training for practitioners in the early years, and parenting programmes, have developed rapidly over the past two decades to incorporate knowledge and understanding of therapeutic support. This approach specifically targets the infant/child's emotional state and coping mechanisms (Bratton et al., 2006; Solihull Approach Parenting Group Research, 2009). The majority of parents will soothe their child effectively and support his emotional regulation. Further positive influences will be gained from a key worker within an early years setting. During these processes, the adult uses containment and supports an infant to acknowledge his emotions, to reflect, and to gain strategies that lessen negative impacts. The infant acquires responses that are embedded within his family culture of values, attitude, and beliefs. The young child will identify feelings and actions with experiences and eventually associate with his regulatory responses. The brain accumulates patterns through the creation of neural networks. These patterns can be regarded as providing a shortcut to infants in their use of protective strategies and resilience that minimises the influence of adversities.

The proximal world of an infant is usually quite narrow, particularly in the earliest days and months of life. The infant's response time to access coping strategies increases as he matures and circumstances and events are experienced on multiple occasions. A sensitive caregiver will instinctively contribute to the child's intentional mental agency by providing a rationale for his emotions and actions, particularly within daily care tasks. An example is gained from the process of nappy changing. An adult responds to the child's emotional and physical discomfort by presenting a practical solution, thus supporting comprehension of intentional mental agency. The child's teleological understanding of a wet sensation followed by parent interaction, and ultimately a dry sensation, is enriched through the merging of his associative emotions and communication strategies. As he matures, the infant begins to use his help-seeking skills proactively in response to his needs. Help-seeking through targeted communication is a key milestone for babies, and there are many opportunities within each day and night for an infant to source responses to his basic physical needs. Parents rapidly gain expertise in interpreting these signals from their baby.

If parents do not demonstrate sensitive responding to the infant, then his sense of self can be adversely affected. Exposure to harm generally activates the attachment system, and infants may seek out physical comfort from caregivers who are abusers. Chaotic disorganised attachment is created. A rise in cortisol levels, as a result of this negative parent-to-child interaction, can result in neuro-developmental abnormalities. The brain's architecture is affected by negative caregiving patterns over time.

A child who is vigilant due to circumstances of perceived danger may demonstrate an increased ability to mentalise his parent's behaviour. This process occurs within, and contributes to, an insecure attachment relationship between child and parent. The infant inherently strives to gain comprehension of his world and to gain a sense of predictability, despite chaotic living conditions. An infant may adopt his parent's negative reactions and assimilate this image internally as his own sense of self. The process results in the child experiencing vulnerability and high anxiety even if he is removed from the source of adversity. His negative representation of himself is stored internally, and led by implicit memories; therefore, the actual source of adversity does not need to be present.

Fonagy (1999) also suggested that children who experienced adversities in early childhood may reject mentalisation of their caregiver's actions. This strategy can provide the child with emotional protection in a context of perceived harm. Alternatively, a mother may not have the capacity to reflect upon her infant's mental state, and instead she dissociates herself from his cries and discomfort. This reaction creates a barrier to the child's understanding of himself through his mother's representation. Inability to use reflective capacity can result in an unstable sense of self in parents and children.

It is thought that negative memories, in a context of childhood abuse, can preside over positive experiences and thereafter increase likelihood of mental-health issues. McCrory et al. (2017) reported that any alteration to threat, reward, and memory-processing could impact upon socialising ability and emotional reactions. These effects could be apparent throughout a lifespan as reaction to new stress is exacerbated.

Transitions

Transitions are particularly significant points of contact. For example, the trau-matised child is entering a service with current experiences of adversity from the home environment affecting his body and mind. A practitioner can set the scene for a child to experience a safe and stimulating session by presenting a positive empathic and nurturing approach. The adult–child relationship supports the child to interpret the physical, emotional, and social learning environment as non-threatening. Short-term negative interactions between peers occur within an early years environment on a daily basis as incremental steps towards social development. For example, sharing and negotiating the use of toys provides numerous opportunities for the practitioner to use the secure attachment rela-tionship to promote positive behaviour and to nurture the child's physiological and emotional regulation.

Children are able to compartmentalise relationships within different envir-onments, and I have often observed insecurely attached children walking quickly away from their parents on entering a service building. The child will focus straight ahead and greet a key worker with positivity. His expectation during this transition is secure attachment to a practitioner in the service. I have noticed some children refusing to turn around or to wave goodbye to a parent despite urgent prompting by the mother or father. Occasionally, a child puts a hand behind his back to wave but remains focused firmly upon the key worker and entrance area of the service. It is fascinating to observe these interactions, and practitioners can gain expertise by seeking out theory and research that extends their comprehension of transitions.

Upon leaving the service, a child will revert to behaviour that he has learned to use in the company of his parent. Environmental factors prompt memories and associated behaviour and actions which the young child has learnt to apply over time. As the proximal context and carers change then the infant demonstrates patterns of behaviour that are based upon emotions. An increase in under-standing the complexities of human relationships by a primary carer contributes to application of supportive strategies in response to each child's needs.

The infant with ambivalent attachment will try a variety of strategies to gain the attention he desires from his parent, for example, holding tightly, hiding his face against a parent, crying for long periods of time, which esca-lates into fear as the parent leaves, and an inability to self-regulate his emo-tions and, consequently, his actions. The timescale of this emotional reaction may be a few minutes or lengthy periods. The high level of anxiety and the direct expression of emotion and needs will subside, and the exhausted child may revert to "still sitting" and non-interaction with the learning environment. The infant or young child's sense of self has been affected negatively. His actions have failed to achieve his desired outcome. Alternatively, this infant may demonstrate aggression towards his parent by rejecting her overtures, removing eye contact, hitting, kicking, and crying angrily. He is expressing negative emotions that are not being met. The infant has an inherent need for consistency and predictability of surroundings and relationships.

Over time, the infant's attachment cues will reduce dramatically if he is not responded to, and avoidant attachment will be demonstrated. The infant will stop attempting to develop an attachment relationship, may appear placid, may remove eye contact from others, may limit his physical explorations, and may begin to demonstrate introverted behaviour. This infant may appear more interested in his own body and clothing as opposed to stimulation within the environment or relationships with others.

Children who have chaotic attachment may experience inconsistent care and neglect that usually includes direct and indirect abuse. Procedural memory, as unconscious memory, is the way in which the child develops expectations of relationships with caregivers which are associated with his patterns of behaviour. These representations can be changed through formal intervention and informal responsive support from an adult, sibling, or peer who nurtures a positive relationship with a child.

The assessment of attachment between parent and child is a challenging area as demonstration of a relationship by a parent and child is influenced by personalities and the culture of a family. Ainsworth established a method of measuring attachment which continues to be used for children aged 12 months. The "Strange Situation" has a focus upon behaviours associated with the stage in which a mother returns to her child after a short absence (Ainsworth et al., 1978). Interactions prior to this age can be measured with the Parent–Infant Observation Scale, the Keys to Interactive Parenting, and the CARE-Index. The Keys to Interactive Parenting review 12 behaviours including limits and consequences (Comfort et al., 2011). The CARE-Index places emphasis upon three aspects of the mother's behaviour towards her child: sensitivity, control, and unresponsiveness, in addition to four aspects of the infant: cooperativeness, compulsivity, difficulties, and passivity (Crittenden, 1985, Crittenden et al., 1991).

Intervention

Howe (2005) identified four different rationale that encompass intervention approaches:

1 Behavioural change in which the parent's sensitivity and responsiveness towards the infant develops.
2 Cognitive change in which the parent's mentalisation of her relationship and behaviour with the child develops.

3   Social change in which the parent is supported to function more effectively through support in a community, home, and alternative environments.
4   Well-being change in which the parent is supported to improve her mental health and physical well-being.

Behavioural change supports a parent to observe her baby or young infant during play and daily routines and to gain knowledge of sleep patterns. The parent learns to view the baby's world, interpreting the environment, stimuli, and relationships from his perspective. The parent learns to notice and to understand his attachment cues and ultimately to develop her capacity to empathise with the baby and to increase her skill of personalised responding.

Cognitive change supports a parent to consider, and to alter, her mentalisation of the parent–child relationship. The parent is encouraged to recall her own childhood experiences. She learns to reflect and to understand the impact of positive *and* negative influences from childhood upon her emotional well-being and desire for learning. Over time, the parent can use this knowledge to alter her understanding of herself and her baby. The parent's attachment model will be reconfigured based upon comparison to past experiences and her hopes and dreams for the baby's future.

Social change supports the parent to gain positive relationships within the home, extended family, and local community. The parent learns to identify appropriate sources of support, to initiate and to develop progressive relationships, and to recognise the positive impact upon her mental health. The parent creates links between her emotional well-being and her parenting abilities.

Well-being change focuses upon support for a parent that increases her physical and mental well-being. Generic intervention by health staff – for example, a midwife and health visitor – provides information and guidance on promoting the well-being of babies and infants. However, it is recognised that the physical well-being of each mother is equally important, pre-birth and post-birth. Physical well-being provides a necessary foundation for mental health to improve and to impact positively upon parenting ability and capacity. An increase in the psychosocial development of a mother has a direct impact upon an attachment relationship and a parent's understanding of intersubjectivity within the parent–child dyad.

Emotions occur as a response to stimuli from the infant's inner working model based upon prior experiences, his instinctive reaction to potential danger, and physiological changes. Emotions also evolve from the infant's reaction to external stimuli in his proximal world. Howe (2005) linked primary carers with psychobiological regulation of an infant's arousal. It is for this reason that interventions should provide opportunities for parents to understand the impact of influences, positive or negative, upon every aspect of the body. Intervention approaches often support a parent's interpretation and understanding from a personal viewpoint but can be enriched by promoting the infant's perspective.

Howe (2005) associated children who have suffered maltreatment with sensory impairment. This researcher uses the terms "clumsy" and "accident-prone" to describe children who have sensory deprivation. Howe indicates that experiences within daily living may cause reactions to trauma which are triggered by an infant recalling a similar incident from his past and by experiencing the associated emotions. This information is based upon sensory input, and it is processed in the limbic system of the brain. The limbic system develops prior to the cognitive areas within the cortex. The infant's instinctive reaction and initial interpretation of stimuli may pose potential threat to his safety and well-being. Practitioners and parents can support reconfiguration of the child's inner working model by nurturing the creation of neural links in cognitive areas of the brain. Plasticity can lead to adaptive patterns of neural networks that respond positively to adversities on a short-term basis; however, research also indicates an increase in vulnerability in later childhood and adulthood.

Every early years practitioner will be able to identify children who react in this way to everyday occurrences, and it is important that practitioners understand and respond sensitively to a traumatised child. Behaviours should be regarded as a complex language, and the practitioner should develop the art of interpreting children's cues and emotional reactions to accurately comprehend their needs. It is not sufficient to provide a nurturing and safe environment to a young, traumatised child in a nursery setting. This child's default position is interpretation of danger until the therapeutic relationship is used to change his understanding. Every single interaction with a child in a setting provides a valuable opportunity to influence his emotions and physiological reactions. Change processes should not only be promoted within the time frame of formal intervention but encompass all aspects of a nursery.

Many nursery activities can be linked to a rationale that promotes the child's resilience, his ability to predict and prepare for outcomes, or to regulate and to contain his emotions in unpredictable circumstances. Examples of hide-and-seek, tig, and peek-a-boo give children an understanding of the permanence of an attachment figure. The infant and young child experience short-term fear in a context of fun, unpredictable actions from the adult and others and the relief and joy of recognising a secure relationship. These games offer fun interactions for both parties in addition to valuable learning opportunities with regard to trust, relationships, and self-regulation of emotions within a short time frame.

Observation and interpretation of the child's body language are the key approach to sensitive responding and to identification of a formal intervention for a family. Body language reveals the child's inner being, which encompasses his physiological and emotional reactions to stimuli. Key aspects to note are frequency of eye contact, verbal or noise communications, movement or non-movement, and the child's stance – standing, sitting, open arms, or body curled up tightly and defensively. A child's use of his hands provides major insight into emotional well-being: fists clenched, hands hidden in pockets or under a blanket, hands used to hide face or specific areas of the body, hands used to protect face or body, hands and arms to comfort self and accompany rocking of the body, hands used for sucking and comfort, hands used to hurt oneself accompanied by direct eye contact and expectation of adult intervention, or non-eye contact and internal focus as the child hurts himself, hands used to actively hit another person or toy or to reject offer of toys, hands used to urgently wave bye in order to reject adult overtures, and open hands and movement of fingers in response to his explorations or interaction from an adult.

I practise child–parent relationship therapy (Bratton et al., 2006), and sessions are used to observe and to gain comprehension of a child's attachment status, his ability, and his capacity to seek out learning from the proximal environment, and to note the impact of prior experiences upon his play. The intervention play and exploration sessions are used to promote and to nurture secure attachment between facilitator and child or parent and child. A popular medium for learning by families, in this context, is the use of videos. The child's emotional well-being and involvement, within this specific learning environment, are assessed and charted by using the Leuven Involvement Scale (Laevers, 1994). These tools provide a means to discuss issues with parents and to clarify comprehension of action, reaction, emotions, and intersubjectivity.

The outcome of therapeutic support is the child's experience of safety within a range of environments, an increased capacity to learn, and an ability to self-regulate his body and mind. Sensory integration experiences can be implemented within interventions and throughout daily routines and play opportunities. Children learn to control their physical bodies and to create links with the accompanying emotions. When physical integration is established then the child begins to understand emotional integration. Sensory-emotional modulation leads to sensory-emotional discrimination, which is promoted through cognitive and language-based therapy, and nurturing approaches to delivery of the curriculum in services. Over time, the child gains insight into his own emotions of despair, anger, guilt, happiness, shame, rage, and fear, which contributes to his increasing understanding of other people's emotions.

Howe (2005) described the processing of emotions at a sensorimotor level and a cognitive level. These processes encompass mental representations and contribute to development of self-regulation. Areas of the brain which are dissociated due to trauma can be integrated by activation of the left cortex and left hemisphere, which deal with language, and the limbic system and right hemisphere, which deal with emotions. Tracking, emotional literacy, and play therapy are informal and formal approaches which are used in early years settings.

During my work with intergenerational families, I observe common patterns in the interactions between parents and children who are insecurely attached. I have noticed that parents in adverse circumstances may pay great heed to the child's physical well-being but ignore emotions. Physical and emotional well-being are partners. Practitioners should use every opportunity to share strategies with parents regarding this significant aspect of development. Parents learn within the context of interventions. Additionally, drop-off and pick-up times in early years settings provide practitioners with opportune circumstances to upskill parents in situ. Emotionally responsive parting and reunions between parents and children create significant developmental blocks that contribute to nurturing a secure attachment relationship. During daily transitions, a key worker can role-model good practice to a parent by describing the child's actions, behaviour, and associative emotions. The practitioner can capitalise upon these opportunities and promote responses that extend a parent's comprehension of the child's physical and emotional well-being.

It is essential to revisit these strategies within a short time period and to reinforce the rationale and skills to the parents. Parents benefit greatly from descriptive praise and recognition from practitioners of their developing skills on this daily informal basis. Learning encompasses every aspect of life, and informal interactions on a nursery doorstep provide ideal circumstances which are conducive to development of parent and child together. These encounters emphasise the importance of working alongside whole families. The ultimate outcome is a secure interdependent family unit whose members support one another to gain resilience to adversities by using their attachment relationships.

Adversities and therapy

Boyce et al. (2021) present factors that influence variation in sibling reaction to adversities. Adversities can be regarded as a lack of supportive conditions for normal development *or* imposition of threatening conditions that disrupt development. Examples include genetic influences, family circumstances, community environments, and developmental timing. This research by Boyce and his colleagues links psychopathology in adulthood to childhood trauma and physiological responses to stress. Unsupportive parenting was identified as influential upon subsequent generations, in addition to undue reactions from participants to their life events. Asmussen et al. (2020) recently published research findings that also indicated negative effects upon the human immune system from lengthy exposure to trauma.

Findings from the research of Boyce et al. (2021) indicated that positive maternal responses can mitigate the negative effects of chronic immune-system activation. This study presented optimum intervention as approaches that are personalised to each child's circumstances and the family context. Inter-agency working is key to implementation as family resources are often depleted in vulnerable families. Intervention must respond to all aspects of life and lifestyle in order to support change and development of children and parents.

A few years ago, I was fortunate to attend a lecture by a visiting relationship counsellor, Charles O'Leary. This educator presented rich information on the practitioner's role in family counselling, and he introduced me to the concept of an "invisible extra beat of time" (O'Leary 2012). The rationale of counselling, regardless of referral criteria, is creating a safe space to think and to talk. It is often the case in early years practice that emphasis is placed upon physical safety due to contexts of child protection and domestic violence. O'Leary emphasised the significance of establishing emotional space to allow freedom of thinking, freedom to remember, to hope, to plan, and to download issues and accompanying emotions.

The extra beat of time reminds the practitioner that his role is to facilitate emotional repair and growth through nurturing resilience to adversity. The early years practitioner cannot remove adversities, but she can support an individual to annul or at least to reduce the impact upon daily living. The practitioner is seeking to understand the other person's perspective and to communicate interest by allocating time. Time is invaluable, but value is not equated to the number of minutes for interactions so much as the quality of space to talk which is created. O'Leary (2012) presented a simplistic but effective gauge to the practitioner: the use of one question demonstrates politeness; the use of two questions demonstrates interest; and the use of three questions demonstrates investment in the other person.

The beat of time within counselling, in a formal or informal context, represents the respect and care that one person has for another. The beat of time can give permission for silence. Silence is required for an individual to absorb the impact of exposing her latent emotions, to embrace physiological changes, and, potentially, to accept her developing relationship overtures that evolve through a counselling session. The beat of time can nurture worthiness, pride, and personal regard in a vulnerable participant.

O'Leary (2012) recommended that the counsellor acknowledges the wisdom of the developing person, and this approach is relevant to early years practice with infants, children, and their parents. Client motivation, quality of relationship, and a client's hope for a positive outcome are cited as contributory factors to change and development. I believe that the quality of relationship can incite motivation for change in parents, and a practitioner's belief in a parent's capacity can ignite hope. Upon reflection on practitioner–parent interactions, I have observed that this belief prompts an actualising tendency. This means that the parent is empowered to change her inner working model and to capitalise upon her skills, strength, and resilience as she progresses along the developmental journey.

The early years practitioner is not usually trained in counselling skills, but he or she has extensive knowledge, understanding, and practical experience in forging, nurturing, and consolidating positive relationships. These relationships, whether practitioner–child or practitioner–parent, provide a necessary foundation for learning and development. Tracking a child's actions, emotions, and intentions is commonplace in a playroom, and the same strategy can provide a useful framework to support parenting skills, formally or informally, at drop-off and pick-up times as described in previous section.

Six conditions for family therapy were promoted widely by O'Leary (2012) and remain applicable to every setting today. These conditions require the practitioner to create an ambient atmosphere, to promote a positive attitude, and, most importantly, to maintain an effective relationship which is enriched by interaction with the developing person. The following section describes these principles in a context of early years practice that relates to formal and informal meetings with families. The practitioner has a role which includes:

1   Seeking to understand and to demonstrate acceptance of each member of the family.
2   Providing a structure for each session.
3   Supporting each family member to identify his or her purpose in the session.

These first three principles present definitive tasks to the early years practitioner from a strategic perspective and practical skill in building relationships for a purpose. It is important to be prepared for a meeting with family members. There have been occasions when I have forgotten to set up the meeting space, and I recall in Box 2.1 a recent example.

Box 2.1 Example from practice

I led a family towards a room which was locked. An old printed black-and-white sign on the closed door declared an identity: Multipurpose Room. For a few seconds, I felt disappointment. I had read this sign many times without due consideration for the message it portrayed to service-users. I wanted the declaration to be vibrant, colourful, attractive, and to set the scene for a welcoming Family Room.

The pencilled time and date in the service booking diary was the only sign of my preparation. I found myself experiencing stress as I realised my failure. I felt anxiety, a dip in confidence, and disappointment in self as I searched frantically for a key, babbling irrelevant excuses as the family waited silently in the darkened corridor. A dusty building smell emanated towards us as I pushed the stiff door with my shoulder to reveal a classic picture of a service meeting room. The old-fashioned metallic blinds were closed, the heating was switched off, and chairs were stacked high in a corner of the room. A stale jug of water sat silently in the middle of the table, a forgotten representation of a previous meeting. The ubiquitous box of tissues lay in waiting at the far side of the table. These circumstances present an immediate barrier to effective information-sharing and interaction.

I tugged the strands of thin nylon cord to open the blinds, and the family helped me to bring forward the cold, plastic chairs. My idea of a semicircle for chatting could not be achieved as I did not want to reject the family's input by rearranging their setting of chairs. My teaching space was smaller than I had planned. The heater sprang into action and created an intrusive hum as the convection setting struggled to impact upon this damp, unwelcoming venue for change.

Preparing a space for a specific purpose demonstrates respect and care for others, and it validates a role for the family and the practitioner. I usually find that families are apprehensive in the initial time period of any meeting, and this emotional reaction may be presented as silence, defensive anger, or disaffection. The first few moments of a conversation sets the atmosphere for family meetings which should be positive and welcoming and present learning in a context of hope for change. As practitioners, we all make mistakes. Distractions divert from preparation, and prioritising needs can impact upon our planned use of time. However, negative environmental issues can be used to the advantage of a positive relationship. Honesty and humility are key levellers in relationships.

I apologised to the family for the lack of preparation. I commented on the cold atmosphere, and we shared laughter as the heater ticked loudly into action. I dramatically threw the stale water away, replacing it with juice and a generous plate of biscuits and encouraging the family to partake. I thanked the family for helping to set our scene for discussion. I confidently moved my chair to create an appropriate and effective learning space between myself and family, explaining my actions. We shared our COVID-19 awareness strategies together, empathising with the challenges and constraints of ever-evolving guidelines. We had established a shared context. The meeting began with positive anticipation.

The final three of O'Leary's principles (O'Leary, 2012) reflect aims for the practitioner to achieve through body language, attitude, and a mindful presence towards interpretation and responses of others.

1   Communicate your belief in each person's ability to actualise her thoughts and wishes.
2   Share knowledge and support change and development.
3   Demonstrate empathy and mindfulness towards the other person.

A positive attitude does not need preparation or to be induced by external props within a meeting space. Belief in another person is conveyed within an attitude that encompasses empathy and personalised care. Listening and considering the other's viewpoints. Observing and reflecting body language, tracking actions, and verbalising emotions from past and present events. Acknowledging and accepting priority of needs as identified by each family member. Contributing the professional perspective, which is led by child protection, knowledge of development, and pedagogy of each service. These relationship skills can be generated from a motivated and confident practitioner in any workspace.

One or multiple interactions with parents can support development of the sense of self in a primary carer. This foundation of knowledge and understanding makes a positive contribution to an infant's mental health by supporting a parent to identify and to make alternative lifestyle choices. The study by Boyce et al. (2021) highlighted the importance of time and neural plasticity to the processes of change and development. This research team also studied emotional regulation and identified that the timing of an intervention was a significant factor in relation to positivity of the child's responses. The degree with which cells and organs are influenced can be used to define their sensitivity to external influences. There are critical and sensitive developmental periods in which plasticity in neural networks facilitates change in response to positive influences.

Genetic and environmental influences

Recent research has shown that genetic and environmental factors can activate, support, or hinder developmental plasticity (Boyce et al., 2021). Mental illness has also been identified as a potential disruptive factor to these processes. These authors found that pathological processes which are associated with some disorders demonstrate the greatest effect before birth and immediately post-birth. Timing is important in nurturing positive effects or minimising negative impact in the interactions of genes, environmental influences, and relationships. The timing of adaptation can affect the outcome. This finding is an important contribution to health promotion and influential to planning and delivery of intervention in the context of disease prevention and the realisation of developmental potential.

Some areas of the brain, for example, circuits which are linked to executive functioning, may continue to be affected by negative influences on a longer-term basis (Boyce et al., 2021; Cross et al., 2017). The work by Asmussen et al. (2020) indicates that *toxic stress* in the early childhood years can result in a reduction of the white matter in the brain that supports executive functioning. This study centred upon Romanian orphanages and, surprisingly, concluded little significant difference in executive functioning of children who experienced foster care and those who remained in institutional care. It may be that the children in orphanages did not experience toxic stress in the form of direct and regular abuse, but a lack of stimulation contributed to weakness in their social, emotional, and cognitive skills. Findings from this research indicated a greater incidence of psychiatric disorders at 12 years of age, and beyond, compared to the norm.

The Bucharest Early Intervention Project researched the emotional development of young children who were placed in foster care following a residential stay in an orphanage (Kondo & Hannan, 2019). Findings indicated that the youngest children, who were less than 2 years old, showed the most positive outcomes for cognitive skill and emotional regulation. It was concluded that cognitive and socio-emotional functions show a high level of adaptation to circumstances during the earliest developmental periods of childhood.

Parents can gain awareness of their contingent responsiveness if they are attuned to their babies' needs. Role-modelling and descriptive praise are useful strategies to support each parent's increase in practical responses which are associated with the baby's emotions. During the first three months of life, babies expect interactions with adults that reflect their emotional states; however, as the baby's interpretation of the world develops, then the interactions can provide appropriate challenges that contribute to development.

The use of video feedback has provided a significant tool in the development of families. It is a familiar medium which society uses to communicate on a daily basis, and it clearly depicts the actions, behaviour, and attitude of a parent in relation to infant's attachment, capacity, and ability to learn and develop. Following an intervention session, I share video feedback with a family, and together we discuss the scenarios that are presented through the recording of interactions between practitioner, parent, and child. Trust, cooperation, and partnership-working can be nurtured through recording and critique of the practitioner's actions and behaviour, which incorporates role-modelling. Subtle but significant gestures, nuances of speech, and overtures of bonding (McClure, 1985) from parent to child can be celebrated and enhanced by sensitive responding.

Behavioural patterns that occur in the earliest weeks and months of life are termed proto-conversational turn-taking. Serve-and-return interactions are important to confirmation of attachment and introduce the wider social and cultural world to the infant. Synchrony may be followed by short instances of rupture and responsive repair. Mid-range tracking and contingency were identified by Beebe and Steele (2013) as repeated patterns of synchrony, rupture, and repair in which the parent effectively regulates herself in addition to her baby. Parental reflective functioning occurs in this context as the primary carer has an awareness of his or her own mental state, the baby's state, and accompanying behaviours. This base of knowledge and understanding requires the parent to acknowledge the infant's capacity to be an intentional mental agent.

Sequencing may not occur if a parent is preoccupied in regulating herself, which may relate to postnatal depression. A parent who is suffering from depression may exhibit low levels of attunement to her baby and lack of synchrony. Alternatively, a mother may demonstrate intensive tracking of the infant in which she imposes control upon his interactions and does not respond to his expressed emotional needs. This parental behaviour is associated with insecure attachment and the parent's representation of the baby as a physical being. These circumstances are often exhibited within my workplace by teenage mothers who are suffering from high levels of anxiety. The parents are seeking to find a sense of an adolescent self, alongside the mothering role.

Box 2.2 Example from practice

I observe a young teenage mother and her new baby attending the service. The baby, mother, and accompanying paraphernalia are clean, and the equipment is in new condition, but the mother is not attuned to her baby's needs. The pram covers are carefully ironed, tucked smoothly and neatly around the little baby, and decorative additions are solely aesthetic for adult viewing as opposed to the baby's comfort. The mother focuses upon showing the pram, bags, bottles, and baby's clothing to practitioners and arranges these artefacts deftly and with pre-planned precision. This young adolescent gives little attention to her baby's emotional state as he copes with the influx of new faces in the vicinity of his world and comfort base, the pram.

His needs at this point in time, and characteristics as a unique and responsive human being, are unheeded by his primary carer. I notice the mother lifting the baby out of the pram and placing him across her shoulder. She automatically faces him away from her view and towards the busy stimulation of urban life. This teenage parent straightens her son's clothing and realigns the presentation of her own outfit as a reaction to the baby wriggling his body in her arms. Eye contact from her baby is not sought by this mother, verbal interaction, and reassurance, supplemented by face-to-face nurturing, and mingling her smell to this little infant's sleep scent is not an observable action during the encounter. Opportunities for secure attachment are available, multifold, but remain disconnected.

I found the research by Lyons-Ruth (2003) interesting as the five behaviours, and apt descriptors which are associated with parental trauma, are observed regularly in the context of parent–infant interaction within a service. The previous practice example depicted these circumstances:

- Threatening: the parent views the baby from above his body and face, which blocks the light and creates an intensive looming presence.
- Dissociative: the parent uses an unusually weak voice which is different to regular communication.
- Deferential or timid: the parent uses a manner of communication that does not instil confidence in a baby, usually through physical interactions.
- Disrupted: the parent does not repair the relationship following periods of rupture.
- Affective communication errors: inappropriate and unpredictable reactions from the parent to the infant's emotions.

A parent's presentation depicts her mental state and capacity at a point in time. Observations at drop-off and pick-up from a service provide invaluable information to use in supporting families to succeed. Early years practitioners interact with parents in the context of childcare sessions within a service. At a surface level, parents may appear to be coping well by arriving on time and attending assiduously to the infant's physical needs. However, multidisciplinary professionals may gain differing views of a parent's well-being and ability to care for a baby which are based upon assessment from the perspective of a particular discipline. For example, health visitors, social workers, and family nurses interact with parents in their home environments.

Living conditions can portray a mother's capacity to embrace, or to be challenged by, motherhood within a daily lifestyle and indicate the level of support from a father and an extended family unit.

During the past year, several pre-birth referrals have been received for our service which describe mothers being hospitalised during the perinatal period due to poor mental health. The research evidence on this significant period, and knowledge of the impact from a mother's well-being to development of her baby, are influencing practice. Reflective functioning can be a complex skill for a mother to acquire if she is coping with mental-health issues. Mental health can reduce the capacity of a mother to observe her child's reactions, to interpret his emotional status, and to use marked mirroring. Depression, anxiety, borderline personality disorders, schizophrenia, domestic violence, substance abuse, parental trauma, and eating disorders can impact negatively upon a parent's health in this context.

Early intervention has to ensure that the parent is healing internally physically, mentally, and emotionally in order that she can focus outwards to her baby's needs from a stable and established sense of self and agency (Miell, 1995). It is important to ascertain physical well-being as the initial step to recovery as mental well-being requires a healthy body as a foundation for emotional healing. Effective practice includes partnership-working by blending the parental and professional expert knowledge of the infant. A practitioner can share information with a primary carer that places great value and worth upon the general parental role but also gives recognition to the characteristics, skills, and preferences of each parent within a specific family culture.

An example of information exchange between professional and parent can include the three wake states for infants termed quiet alert, unsettled, and crying. Additionally, the three sleep states are described as drowsy, light, or deep sleep. In the early days of a baby's life, his parents will focus assiduously on sleep and wake patterns. Every conversation enlightens a listener upon the number of hours of sleep which a parent has achieved, and is often linked to a judgement of a "good" baby. I find that parents have acute insight into their babies' patterns of behaviour throughout each day and night, but it is often the case that parents do not appreciate the significance and value of this knowledge. A reflective practitioner will prompt a parent to share this knowledge through direct questions, professional curiosity, and demonstration of a desire to create an integrated partnership with an infant's primary carers.

All babies will experience these six states throughout each day, but, over time, wake/sleep patterns are established that can be associated with routines and expectations within each family. For example, parents can encourage progress from drowsy to deep sleep through a bedtime routine, and in the early hours of daylight the baby can be supported sensitively to transition from a light sleep state to quiet alert in preparation for his first feed.

Nurturing environment

Services may focus upon delivering universal, targeted, or indicated approaches in relation to service rationale, funding opportunities, and needs in the local area. Engaging parents in an intervention is a key issue (Edelman, 2004), and non-engagement is a barrier to development of mother and child. Consideration should be given to parent's learning styles, motivation, and social ability to interact in group or individual support sessions. Informal universal approaches incorporate aspects of targeted and indicated interventions. For example, empowerment of parents to support realisation of inherent parenting skills and promoting the sense of self and the agency of the mother/father and child (Heath, 2004).

A recently published study by Fukkink (2021) reviewed the well-being of children aged 0–4 years within day care. Findings indicated that well-being varied significantly throughout the day for each child in the participant sample of 30; however, the average recording of well-being in this study was defined as neutral. The researcher described this finding as well-being without dominant signs of joy or discomfort. Links were made between well-being and free-play or teacher-led activities as opposed to lower well-being during transitions, mealtimes, and peer conflicts. The data did not indicate an association between a child's well-being and a carer's sensitivity. Recommendations highlighted the need for carers to respond quickly to the socio-emotional needs of infants due to rapid fluctuation of well-being within a day-care setting.

Creating a COVID-safe environment in services has presented challenges; however, many measures have positive, and unexpected, outcomes. At entry to a service, the infant is introduced to a key worker and led gently away from the parent or carried into a playroom to commence the transition period while parents complete necessary paperwork. Surprisingly, young children have been adapting to the service more quickly and positively without their parents being present in the playroom. The key worker is the secure attachment figure in the early stages, and the increase in stimulation and a nurturing environment in addition to therapeutic pedagogy are key factors in facilitating this transition.

The use of contingent responsiveness, role-modelling, prompting, scaffolding, and interpretation of each child's mental health by marked mirroring are supportive strategies to inclusion and attainment. A baseline is created to support progress throughout childhood and beyond (Bomber, 2007; Department for Children, Schools and Families, 2010; Geddes, 2006). Parents have accepted the COVID-safe conditions, and photographs, videos, and regular feedback by phone or social media reassure families that their children are well and thriving in the nursery environment.

Trevarthen (2001) used the term "relation emotions" to identify emotions that are associated with companionship and separate from self-regulatory emotions. Examples of the self-regulatory emotions refer to experiences of pain, pleasure, or hunger. This research study indicated that relation emotions are associated with mental illness through a lack of intersubjectivity. Sroufe et al.

(2000) described negative impacts upon interpersonal relationships as potential criteria for a diagnosis of psychopathology and a route to understanding the origin of this disorder in adulthood. Experience of negative parenting techniques in the form of rejection, or lack of supervision, are deemed to be risk factors for the child developing psychopathology in later life. Emotional unavailability is associated with conduct problems in childhood and may be contextualised by parental disharmony and violence. The research indicated the significance of relationships to human functioning. Positive, secure, and consistent relationships can reduce the negative impacts. However, this research also raised the issue of "boundary violation". This term was used by the authors in reference to a parent interacting with the infant in a similar relationship to the peer or spouse partnership (Sroufe et al., 2000).

The research by Condon and Corkindale (2011) on antenatal attachment had a participant group of 238 women in their third trimester of pregnancy. Findings indicated that depression and a lack of social support are detrimental to the mother's attachment to her baby prior to birth. Additionally, antenatal attachment was suggested as an indicator for maternal infant attachment. This research described relationships as encompassed by interconnections and emotional regulation that can be linked to psychopathological disorders. Condon and Corkindale (2011) concluded in their study that services should respond to an expectant mother's low mood and limitations in social support from extended family or friends during the antenatal period. The significance of intervention before birth is related to the development of secure attachment after birth. Sroufe et al. (2000) found that alternative relationships to primary carer and child were also effective in minimising the negative impact of adversity, for example links to grandparents or a therapist.

During the first year of life, an infant learns to adapt his responses in accordance with the reactions or lack of responsive action by his primary carer. For example, a distressed infant may lift his arms above his head and cry for support; however, if the support is not forthcoming, then he will learn to take further action and to crawl towards an adult. Sroufe et al. (2000) describe this stage as the infant progressing from the use of reflexive signalling to active intentional communication. These infantile foundations are essential to support comprehension of the autobiographical self, and secure attachment within a dyadic relationship facilitates the processes. Furthermore, relationships in middle childhood and adolescence will evolve positively if the capacity and ability for self-regulation has been realised in infanthood.

It is known that the interplay of genes, environment, and time promote a unique response in each child, and subsequent actions and outcomes are also influenced by personality. Boyce et al. (2021) emphasised the impact of genetic variation upon the individual's sensitivity to adversity, and to trauma, and this study cited a lack of supportive parenting as increasing these risks. The research indicated a causal element to risk as sympathetic activation of inflammatory cytokine production. Family support that promotes strengths and supports weaknesses is promoted as an effective intervention.

Interestingly, the research by Boyce et al. (2021) included a study of the adolescent period, and findings suggested that maternal responsivity can protect against or reduce the impact from chronic immune system activation. The period of growth in the teenage years is regarded as a time when cells and organs are sensitive and reactive to external influences. The researchers referred to differential plasticity through comparison of sensory processing which can respond to influences within months, and executive functioning which can be responsive to external influences throughout the lifespan. As critical period timing varies in individuals, it not only exposes challenges for the implementation of intervention but also increases opportunities for change and development.

Humans are predisposed to seek relationships and interactions with others from birth and to share their emotional reactions to the external environment, in addition to expressing their internal states through behaviour. The infant is immersed in family and community culture, which affects his understanding and interactions with the world from birth. Svanberg and Barlow (2009) identify significant aspects of an infant's emotional development between one and six months:

- His capacity to use reciprocal interactions with caregivers.
- His experience of a range of emotional states.
- His need for containment.
- His development of an early representation of his sense of self, and others.
- His cognitive and intellectual growth.
- The level of his parents' sensitivity and responsiveness.

The research by Davis and Montag (2019) described the use of emotions in mammals as fulfilling the need for survival, to nurture young, and to encourage participation and interaction with a stimulating learning environment. Early experiences create patterns for the creation of future relationships and a foundation for self-regulation of emotions and behaviour. Sroufe et al. (2000) linked effective self-regulation in adulthood with experience gained within an adult–child dyad during the earliest years.

Barlow and Svenberg (2009) highlighted that a negative impact upon an infant can be expressed through neglect or intrusion by a mother who is experiencing depression and low mental health. The infant experiences disruption periods of inconsistent attention and lack of attention, and there may also be periods of positive interaction with a primary carer. These babies may develop insecure attachment in the early stages of life and learn to up-regulate in a bid to gain attention and down-regulate as a self-protection strategy over time. The babies acquire behaviours in response to their mothers' changing moods, abilities, and capacity to provide care.

Research has indicated that a parent's mind-mindedness, as used by Barlow and Svenberg (2009) in depicting a parent's sensitive responding to her child's needs and emotions, is a more effective predictor of developmental rate than educational background or socio-economic status. Beebe and Steele (2013) identified that the infant's experiences guide his perception of himself, in addition to development of strategies to deal with negative emotions, and this is influenced by interactions with his primary carer. In a context of danger, the young child may be hypervigilant and more acutely aware of his mother's cues in relation to his internal mental state. Fonagy (1999) describes a mother presenting her child with a particular mental state through actions and behaviour in response to his needs. This author regarded reflective capacity as a transgenerational acquisition.

It is also indicated that the infant in adverse circumstances has greater capacity to interpret the mental state of his primary carer than his own mental state. A mother may reflect, and consequently exacerbate, the negative emotions of the infant or ignore his state of stress. The study by Cassidy and Mohr (2006) indicated a status which was termed as unsolvable fear. The authors expressed that it appeared impossible for an infant to develop organised attachment responses within a context of a chronic source of fear.

Cassidy (1994) explored the close links between attachment relationships and the ability and capacity to regulate emotions in infanthood. Infants who have avoidant attachment, through rejection by a primary carer, will minimise emotional impact by actively reducing their relationship cues as a protective strategy. These actions are described by Cassidy as contributory to maintaining the parent's own state of mind in which the need for attachment is minimised. Alternatively, infants who have developed ambivalent attachment through intermittent availability of a primary carer will use a variety of means to capture attention. These actions represent the infant's need for an attachment relationship and directly influence the parent's responses to attachment cues.

Underdown (2009) identified touch as a powerful and effective tool in creating and sustaining a secure attachment relationship between mother and child. This author indicated that lack of tactile connection adversely affected emotional development and physical health and growth. The use of infant massage, as a learned intervention, has increased greatly since McClure founded the International Association of Infant Massage in the United States (McClure, 1985). Infant massage reduces and stabilises cortisol, epinephrine, and norepinephrine, which relate to the level of stress experienced by a baby or child (Underdown, 2006).

A child with disorganised attachment may experience historical ideas and emotions with the same intensity as current external events. Parents often express that their children "are reliving past experiences" in a context of trauma and child abuse. Practitioners observe children in nurseries immersed in thought and outwardly exhibiting signs of internal stress, for example, sucking clothing, twisting hands together, biting lips, or clenching fists. Insecure relationships during infancy may lead to personality distortions in later stages of development as described by Fonagy (1999).

An interesting study by Witherington and Crichton (2007) focuses upon the functionalist approach to emotions. These authors describe the emotion system as a complex nonlinear system that functions in accordance with interaction of the components. Development in one area can alter the system, for example, motor skill and the accompanying emotions. The authors indicate that behaviour by an infant is influenced by emotional reaction and used to establish, to maintain, or to change the relationship with a proximal environment. An example of a new skill is crawling and venturing beyond the Circle of Security in relation to a primary carer. This gross motor skill may incur fear or excitement and achievement; thus, the emotion system is reconfigured based upon an increase in knowledge, understanding, and potentially new interpretation of the world. The reconfiguration reflects an impact of emotions as the infant explores, learns, and develops.

A recent publication from the UK Government (2021) describes an impactful intervention as the Healthy Child Programme in England. It is a national public-health framework for children and young people. Health promotion is available from birth to 19 years, or 25 if the young person has particular health needs. Antenatal, newborn, and infant screening for health issues are also encompassed within the delivery of this programme. NHS England provide a postnatal check for new mothers and their babies at 6 to 8 weeks, which includes mental health and well-being of the mother.

References

Ainsworth, M. D. S., Blehar, M. C., Waters, E., & Wall, S. (1978). *Patterns of attachment: A psychological study of the Strange Situation.* Hillsdale, NJ: Erlbaum.

Asmussen, K., Fischer, F., Drayton, E., & McBride, T. (2020). Adverse childhood experiences: What we know, what we don't know, and what should happen next. https://www.eif.org.uk/report/adverse-childhoodexperiences-what-we-know-what-we-dont-know-and-what-should-happen-next.

Association of Infant Mental Health, UK. (2021). The infant mental health competency framework. https://aimh.uk/the-uk-imh-competency-framework.

Barlow, J., & Svenberg, P. O. (2009). Keeping the baby in mind. In J. Barlow & P. O. Svanberg (Eds.), *Keeping the baby in mind: Infant mental health in practice* (pp. 1–16). Hove: Routledge.

Beebe, B., & Steele, M. (2013). How does microanalysis of mother–infant communication inform maternal sensitivity and infant attachment? *Attachment & Human Development*, 5(5–6),583–602.

Bomber, L. M. (2007). *Inside I am hurting: Practical strategies for supporting children with attachment difficulties in schools.* London: Worth.

Bowlby, J. (1979). *The making and breaking of affectional bonds.* Abingdon and New York: Routledge.

Boyce, W. T., Levitt, P., Martinez, F. D., McEwen, B. S., & Shonkoff, J. P. (2021). Levaraging the biology of adversity and resilience to transform pediatric practice. *Pediatrics*, 147(2): e20201651.

Bratton, S. C., Landreth, G. L., Kellam, T., & Blackard, S. R. (2006). *Child/parent participation therapy treatment manual.* Abingdon and New York: Routledge.

Cassidy, J. (1994). Emotion regulation: Influences of attachment relationships. *Monograph Social Residential Child Development*, 59 (2–3),228–249.

Cassidy, J., & Mohr, J. (2006). Unsolvable fear, trauma, and psychology: Theory, research and clinical considerations related to disorganised attachment across the life span. *Clinical Psychology: Science and Practice*, 8(3), 275–298.

Comfort, M., Gordon, P. R., & Naples, D. (2011). KIPS: An evidence-based tool for assessing parenting strengths and needs in diverse families. *Infants and Young Children*, 24(*1*), 56–74.

Condon, J. T., & Corkindale, C. (2011). The correlates of antenatal attachment in pregnant women. *British Journal of Medical Psychology*, 70(*4*), 359–372.

Cooper, G., Hoffman, K., & Powell, B. (2016). The Circle of Security. https://www.circleofsecurityinternational.com/circle-of-security-model/wha t-is-the-circle-of-security.

Crittenden, P. M. (1985). Maltreated infants: vulnerability and resilience. *Journal of Child Psychology and Development*, 26, 85–96.

Crittenden, P. M., Partridge, M. F., & Claussen, A. H. (1991). Family patterns of relationship in normative and dysfunctional families. *Development and Psychopathology*, 3(*4*), 491–512.

Cross, D., Fani, N., & Powers, A. (2017). Neurobiological development in the context of childhood adversity. *Clinical Psychological Science Practice*, 24, 111–124.

Davis, K. L., & Montag, C. (2019). Selected principles of Pankseppian affective neuroscience. *Frontiers in Neuroscience*, 12(1025).

Department for Children, Schools and Families. (2010). *Breaking the link between disadvantage and low achievement in the early years: Everyone's business.* Nottingham: Department for Children, Schools and Families.

Department of Health and Social Care. (2021). The best start for life: A vision for the 1001 critical days. Policy paper. https://www.gov.uk/government/publications/the-best-start-for-life-a-vision-for-the-1001-critical-days.

Douglas, H., & Rheeston, M. (2009). The Solihull Approach: An integrative model across agencies. In J. Barlow & P. O. Svanberg (Eds.), *Keeping the baby in mind: Infant mental health in practice* (pp. 29–39). Hove: Routledge.

Doyle, C. (2001). Surviving and coping with emotional abuse in childhood. *Clinical Child Psychology and Psychiatry*, 6 (*3*). London: Routledge.

Edelman, L. (2004). A relationship-based approach to early intervention. http//www.cde.state.co.us/earlychildhoodconnections/Technical.htm.

Farmer, E., & Owen, M. (1995). *Child protection practice: Private risks and public remedies.* London: HMSO.

Fonagy, P. (1999). Transgenerational consistencies of attachment: A new theory. *Dallas Society for Psychoanalytic Psychology.* http://www.dspp.com/papers/fonagy2.htm.

Fukkink, R. G. (2021). Exploring children's wellbeing in day-care: How do children feel all day? *European Early Childhood Education Research Journal.* https://doi.org/10.1080/1350293X.2021.2007971.

Geddes, H. (2006). *Attachment in the classroom: The links between children's early experience, emotional wellbeing, and performance in school.* London: Worth.

Heath, H. (2004). Assessing and delivering parent support. In M. Hoghughi & N. Long (Eds.), *Handbook of parenting theory and research for practice* (pp. 315–322). London: Sage.

Howe, D. (2005). *Child abuse and neglect: Attachment, development, and intervention.* Basingstoke: Palgrave Macmillan.

Kondo, M. A., & Hannan, A. J. (2019). Environmental stimulation modulating the pathophysiology of neurodevelopmental disorders. In L. M. Oberman & P. G. Enticott (Eds.), *Neurotechnology and Brain Stimulation in Pediatric Psychiatric and Neurodevelopmental Disorders* (pp. 31–54). Elsevier Academic Press.

Laevers, F. (1994). *Defining and assessing quality in early childhood education*. Leuven: Leuven University Press.

Levine, A., Zagoory-Sharon, O., Feldman, R., & Weller, A. (2007). Oxytocin during pregnancy and early postpartum: individual patterns and maternal-fetal attachment. *Peptides, 28(6)*, 1162–1169.

Lyons-Ruth, K. (2003). The two-person construction of defenses: Disorganized ... /helpless relational processes. *Journal of Infant Child and Adolescent Psychotherapy* 2(4), 105–114.

Maslow, A. (2000). Maslow's hierarchy of needs. *Encyclopedia of Personality and Individual Differences*. https://www.semanticscholar.org/paper/Maslow%E2%80%99s-Hierarchy-of-Needs-Maslow/7eba323b291188524755a7cc0bda63aaba9c5abd.

McClure, V. (1985). *Infant massage: A handbook for loving parents*. New York: Bantam Books.

McCrory, E. J., Gerin, M. I., & Viding, E. (2017). Childhood maltreatment, latent vulnerability, and the shift to preventative psychiatry: The contribution of functional brain imaging. *Journal of Child Psychology, 58(4)*, 338–357.

Miell, D. (1995). The development of self. In P. Barnes (Ed.), *Personal, social and emotional development of children* (pp. 190–201). Blackwell: Open University.

O'Leary, C. J. (2012). *The practice of person-centred couple and family therapy*. Basingstoke: Palgrave Macmillan.

Royal College of Midwives (2020). Parental emotional wellbeing and infant development. https://www.rcm.org.uk/media/4645/parental-emotional-wellbeing-guide.pdf.

Solihull Approach Parenting Group Research. (2009). Solihull approach parenting group research and NICE guidelines. https://solihullapproachparenting.com/research.

Sroufe, A., Duggal, S., Weinfield, N., & Carlson, E. (2000). Relationships, development, and psychopathology. In A. J. Sameroff, M. Lewis, & S. M. Miller *Handbook of developmental psychology*, 2nd edition (pp. 75–91). New York: Kluwer Academic/Plenum Publishers.

Svanberg, P. O., & Barlow, J. (2009). Developing infant centred services: The way forward. In J. Barlow & P. O. Svanberg (Eds.), *Keeping the baby in mind: Infant mental health in practice* (pp. 185–198). Hove: Routledge.

Tomasello, M. (1999). The human adaptation for culture. *Annual Review Anthropology, 28*, 509–529.

Trevarthen, C. (2001). Intrinsic motives for companionship in understanding: Their origin, development, and significance for infant mental health. *Infant Mental Health Journal, 22(1–2)*,95–131.

Underdown, A. (2006). *Young children's health and well-being*. Maidenhead: McGraw Hill/Open University Press.

Underdown, A. (2009). Keeping the baby in mind. In J. Barlow & P. O. Svanberg (Eds.), *Keeping the baby in mind: Infant mental health in practice* (pp. 17–28). Hove: Routledge.

UNICEF. (2021). Baby friendly initiative. https://www.unicef.org.uk/babyfriendly/baby-friendly-resources/implementing-standards-resources/skin-to-skin-contact.

Witherington, D. C., & Crichton, J. A. (2007). Frameworks for understanding emotions and their development: Functionalist and dynamic systems' approaches. *Emotion, 7(3)*, 628–637.

3 The developing child

Chapter 3 reviews developmental processes and includes discussion on the developing sense of self in the earliest years. Mitigating factors are described as the psychological resources of each adult, personality, and particular characteristics of an infant. Sroufe et al. (2000) indicated that infants have the ability to adjust their behaviour if an adult misinterprets the initial cues. Asmussen et al. (2020) advised that adversities may incur deprivation of intellectual stimulation. Overcoming this detrimental effect requires particular adaptation by a child, and this chapter explores high ability (Silverman, 2016), internal and external asynchrony, and additional needs.

Knowledge and understanding from flow theory are used to describe influences upon development which include situational features and personal characteristics (Csikszentmihalyi, 1990). The six conditions of a therapeutic relationship by Rogers (1990) are also presented to the reader for consideration. Rogers had stated that specialist knowledge is not required in the creation of a therapeutic relationship. Differentiation is made between the concepts of caring for someone that encompasses physical, and environmental care or caring about someone that refers to a carer's responses to needs, and emotional reactions (Hogg & Warne, 2010).

Attainment gap

I consider an infant's chronological age and his stages of development, which are led by interaction of gene potential and environmental factors. This knowledge identifies contributory factors to the expansion of an attainment gap between the average child and disadvantaged children. Babies and toddlers who attend my workplace struggle to cope with daily survival, and withdrawal symptoms are common from birth to 18 months due to parental drug or alcohol use. These adversities can be experienced directly from mother to foetus or indirectly from both parents using drugs within the home environment. Asmussen et al. (2020) recently expressed that further research is required to gain understanding of the social processes that prolong the impact of adversities, in addition to the emotional aspects that increase a child's resilience. All topics are complimentary to one another within the context of infant mental health.

DOI: 10.4324/9781003358107-3

Research indicates that babies can experience internal states in relation to seeking support, rage, fear, pain, loss, play, and care. These emotions contribute to the infant's or child's developing sense of self over time. Activation of a baby's emotions results in physiological change, for example cortisol release, and subsequently impacts upon behaviour. An infant's interpretation of the world can be led by the primary carer's reaction, or the key worker's, in the circumstances of a child attending services. Young children's emotional literacy can easily be supported within daily living. The early stages of self-regulation can be initiated through sensitive care that supports up-regulation and promotes a pathway to down-regulation if responses are paced appropriately to personality and needs. Therapeutic intervention can be used to identify and to respond to developmental gaps by increasing knowledge and skills of the child, parent, and practitioner. I have always taught the concepts of self and agency in partnership, which increases understanding of these issues to practitioners.

The term "marking", in relation to mirroring, refers to a parent, or practitioner in a service, responding to a child by copying his emotions initially and subsequently presenting an interpretation of a situation for the child to assimilate. By using this approach, an adult can nurture a child's skill of independent emotional containment. Infants reflect the emotions of a parent which can be prohibitive of positive emotional development if the parent is suffering from short- or long-term mental-health issues.

Box 3.1 Example from practice

Nine-month-old Murad and his mother, Ebi, have recently commenced nursery. It is clear that Murad is aware of the sudden increase in noise and stimulation in his personal space. During lockdown periods, he had a quiet, predictable lifestyle at home with his mother and older brother. Murad is seated comfortably on a thick, woollen, red-checked rug in which each square is adorned with a farm animal – cows, sheep, chickens, and horses dance across the rug ready to stimulate little learners. However, Murad does not feel comfortable. He glances from side to side without moving his body. His fists are clenched and held tightly against his body. I have often observed children hiding their hands during periods of anxiety. A fire engine suddenly creates a raucous intrusion as this external influence impinges upon the ambience of the nursery playroom.

The key worker and Ebi are seated on a navy corner settee, under a dark-green canopy which is strewn with artificial greenery and flowers: the book corner and nurture area. The practitioner is completing induction forms, seeking permission from Murad's primary carer for the nursery team to take the little boy outside the building, to change his nappy, to brush his teeth, to participate in individual play, to take photographs, and many more examples that encompass a typical nursery day.

Murad makes a plaintive whimper of fear, his cry is directed randomly outwards as he is unable to see his mother seated within the nurture corner. The key worker smiles and quickly gestures to Ebi to approach her son. The induction forms are deprioritised in preference to the infant's needs. Ebi kneels beside Murad. Her large mother-and-baby bag slides forward from her shoulder, and impatiently she pushes it aside. This mother has one focus only at this moment: responding to Murad's emotion. I notice that momentarily Ebi mimicked the infant's distressed face, and she acknowledged her son's angst by expressing his negative emotion to him verbally. However, a reassuring hand upon his back, a mother's broad smile, nodding with positivity, and using motherese to create a non-threatening atmosphere supported Murad to regain his composure.

In a few moments, this little child leant against his mother, his mouth uplifted in a smile, and he nodded up and down as his relaxing body demonstrated liberation from potential threat and fear. I commented to this mother on the effect of her skills, I described her actions, and I linked to Murad's self-esteem and regaining of his composure: marked mirroring. Ebi shrugged as she looked down shyly, seemingly embarrassed to receive my recognition. I said her name clearly, and, as this young mother looked up, I reiterated my message, "Ebi, you are the expert on your child's needs. I want to learn from you on how to support Murad to achieve." This time Ebi nodded, and I could see that she felt pleased and perhaps empowered.

Similar momentary incidents occur frequently within every early years service and in a home environment. I often observe marked mirroring from mother to child upon public transport on my journey home from work. I feel strongly that practitioners and parents should be given awareness of the value of their input to a distressed infant. The interaction may appear to be insignificant, and a natural response, but it contributes to an essential foundation for development of a sense of self and regulation of emotions. Senior staff and key workers should gain confidence in noticing and tracking each other's practice and by reaffirming through verbal recognition. Early years practitioners should capitalise upon opportunities to give parents positive feedback on parenting skills, within and out-with interventions.

Trauma impacts upon the comprehension of one's own mind and subsequently upon the capacity to appreciate the mind of a baby. Mirroring without marking can also occur between parent and child. A mother who has unresolved trauma replicates and emphasises the infant's own reaction without emotional containment. The infant is not presented with an understanding of his emotions in relation to context or supported to develop resilience, or to adopt social behaviours. Alternatively, the parent's own emotion which is based upon implicit memories of historical trauma may be communicated and adopted by the infant. The former response can prolong the trauma reaction, and the latter contributes to the baby's creation of a false sense of self.

An infant can develop a false sense of self by referring to interpretation of the world from another person's perspective and by adopting their emotional reactions. His representation of the world is a direct copy from his role model, as opposed to his emotions and behaviour being influenced by experiential learning. At times, parents may contribute inadvertently to this dependency by directing the child's actions and dismissing his cues. Montessori (1964) promoted the key-worker system in services and elevated the significance of the role of primary carer to secure attachment figure in the earliest years of childhood. Siraj-Blatchford et al. (2003) researched the effects from multiple carers on children's development in a long-term study called The Effective Provision of Pre-school Education Project (Department for Education and Skills, 2004). Findings reported positive effects from the consistent care of a key worker and professional–parent relationships. This approach to nurturing children in services continues throughout the world. A responsibility of the key worker is promotion of each infant's sense of self and agency.

The use of containment encompasses the delivery of intervention in a service (Bratton et al., 2006) and supports the skill of reflective functioning. It is essential that practitioners communicate comprehension of these processes to each parent in response to individual modes of learning, for example, by using video feedback to prompt discussion and reflection upon the parent's actions and baby's responses. The aforementioned child–parent relationship therapy is filmed at each session and used to increase understanding of parent and practitioner.

Many countries have placed an increase in emphasis on supporting practitioners, in a breadth of disciplines, to gain knowledge and practical expertise in the field of infant mental health. My workplace is informed by the recent Scottish framework for practice that promotes understanding from the impact of trauma upon neurological, biological, psychological, and social development (Scottish Government & NHS Scotland, 2021). There are five key principles:

1 Physical and emotional safety.
2 Transparency and trustworthiness.
3 Choices and voice.
4 Collaboration and development.
5 Empowerment of individual and organisations.

The projected result is an increase in positive responses to service-users who are affected by adversity, in addition to nurturing self-compassion in the workforce and leading to an improvement in mental health for all.

A sense of self

By five years of age, most children have developed an elementary sense of the autobiographical self by experiencing five consecutive stages of learning (Whitters, 2018).

1   Physical agency.
2   Social agency.
3   Teleological agency.
4   Intentional agency.
5   Representational agency.

These stages are traversed incrementally, and development is iterative in relation to experiences and opportunities for learning based upon an infant's personal interests. This responsive context maintains a high level of involvement with the environment and nurtures emotional well-being. As I previously commented, the average age of a sense of self emerging (Stern 1998) differs markedly from my experience of an infant's comprehension of his emergent, core, subjective, and verbal self, in contexts of adversity. The negative effects of adverse childhood influences upon the timing of the stages of normative development are clear. These milestones represent the infant's growing sense of agency in which he understands and uses his ability, and capacity to influence the environment and people. Trauma can delay or prevent the child's comprehension of agency progressing. Psychopathological disorders are linked to gaps in functioning within these states of agency.

During the first year of life, an infant will begin to demonstrate intentional actions. He has elementary understanding of cause and effect: for example, lifting both arms towards his parent is a direct cue for a nurturing response. If this action is rewarded by close physical contact that supports his emotional need, then the infant will quickly learn patterns of cause and effect as responses to his physiological and emotional experiences.

The work of Sroufe et al. (2000) showed that infants have the ability to adjust their behaviour if an adult misinterprets the initial cues. For example, the action of raising both arms might be extended to include fists opening and closing, indicating that the child is seeking to latch onto his parent. Over time, these early experiences will be used by the infant to generalise beyond the care of his mother or father, and his expectations of action and reaction will be extended to other adults and, potentially, siblings. Sroufe et al. (2000) describe attachment as the dyadic regulation of emotions in infants which is operationalised by the caregiver guiding the young child's self-regulation. Caregivers have an essential role in providing a child with opportunities to regulate his emotions through the use of predictable, consistent responses to his needs and actions. Over time, the infant's inner working model retains this increase in knowledge and understanding.

Memory, and actions associated with secure attachment in early childhood, directly influence the capacity and ability to create positive and fulfilling relationships in middle childhood, adolescent years, and adulthood. Sroufe et al. (2000) link insecure attachment to anxiety disorders, dissociative symptoms, which can be associated with chaotic circumstances, and inconsistent relationships during childhood, but not causally. Psychopathology results from combinations of multiple adverse influences and lack of protective factors throughout the lifespan.

Gaining insight into normal learning and developmental processes provides a route for intervention to facilitate and to support systems for infants who have been adversely affected by internal and external influences. In the earliest stages, following birth, the infant demonstrates a propensity for his mother's voice which has been a consistent circumstantial aspect throughout his growth period in utero. Newly born babies also indicate a desire to seek out their mother's eye contact, recognise her appearance within a few days, and react positively to maternal smell as opposed to the smell of other adults. Trevarthen and Aitken (2001) describe evidence of 6-month-old infants who were motivated to share cognition with caregivers that related to their proximal environment. During the first year of life, an infant demonstrates a range of emotions that encapsulate his desire to engage with learning.

Box 3.2 Example from practice

Xiang is six months and started nursery today. Six months is a useful age to commence a service as most children are ready to accept a second attachment figure in their quest for knowledge and understanding of a widening world. The new baby's parents had been relieved when their daughter had finally arrived. Nine months of hopes and dreams had culminated in a beautiful raven-haired girl whose tiny nails were bright pink, and her cheeks flushed red as she entered the world. On arrival at nursery, Xiang did not cling to her key worker for reassurance, but the infant moved her head around and about as she noticed the new environment. Xiang activated her senses quickly to absorb this increase in stimulation.

Xiang had managed to sit independently from 4 months of age, and currently, at 6 months, she could balance with a straight back, reach for toys, resume a sitting stance, and competently transfer items from one hand to another. This skill contributes to the creation of a baseline for exploration and supports acquisition of immense knowledge in the first year of life. Xiang's fingers worked in tandem to turn over a fir cone, her tongue and lips confirmed the hard properties of this natural object, and her nose detected a similar smell to home as the cone had been cleaned industriously with disinfectant by a member of staff. Her eyes observed the item from every angle, and her ears messaged no sound from shaking the fir cone.

Xiang sought eye contact with her key worker, seeking a reference point for her investigations. The explorer paused for a few seconds as the key worker responded to her cues for interaction and conversed with the 6-month-old infant. Xiang sat very still for a few seconds as she listened and absorbed information from this new voice which would quickly become a familiar backdrop to nursery. Moments later, Xiang discarded the item in a definitive backward throw, but, interestingly, the young learner swivelled around, and she attempted to retrieve her chosen toy. Only infants can turn successfully in a complete circle by using their legs as rudders and bodies as ballast. Learning opportunities emerge in vast quantities when this 360-

degree motor skill is achievable. Xiang's memory was certainly active, and her neural connections were rapidly creating a vivid picture to inform her inner working model. A smile enveloped Xiang, and her head bobbed up and down as she demonstrated great motivation to engage with the learning environment of her nursery playroom and to commence a relationship with her key worker.

Emotions and communication

Babies exhibit communication cues continuously, and time to observe is essential within a nursery environment and the home. When any adult approaches a baby then it is important to take a few seconds to assess the infant's circumstances, emotions, and involvement with the proximal environment. An adult should aim to seamlessly create a dyad with an infant that compliments and takes account of his current status, including his physiological well-being, his emotional reaction to the adult's presence, and his immediate interests. A necessary first stage to development is comprehending and accommodating the young child's reaction and interaction to his world prior to a dyad being formed.

Plutchik (1980) investigated emotions in infants, and the study indicated that emotions were organised in a similar way within adults and young children. A few years later, Panksepp (1998) identified opposing pairs of emotions that related to basic functions for survival and regulation of behaviour: seeking/curiosity, fear/escape, rage/attack, and distress/affection.

An obvious desire to learn which is accompanied by emotion can act as a source of motivation for a parent to engage in an intersubjective dyad with the infant in a context of imitative and complementary reciprocal responses. This aspect of development contributes to daily living within a family and community culture. However, dis-regulation of such emotions can indicate psychological disorders, including difficulties in relating to objects and people (Trevarthen & Aitken, 2001).

An awareness of the permanence of meaning, as termed by Trevarthen and Aitken (2001), is also acquired within the first 12 months of childhood, and the infant apportions intrinsic value to particular gestures and resultant actions. These communications are often immersed within the family culture or relevant to a particular caregiver. Maternal or paternal depression affects operational skills in daily living and impacts upon relationships with others. The creation of positive relationships can create a foundation for intervention and a means to repair the adverse effects.

Parenting role

Belsky (1984) identified three domains which affect the parenting role.

1 The psychological resources of each adult.
2 Personality and particular characteristics of each child.
3 The environmental context of stress and the minimising or maximising factor of support.

This author expressed that the capacity and ability of the parent is the most significant factor. It is often the case that concerns about attachment are expressed as a child not having secure attachment to an adult. Each infant has an inherent predisposition to seek out positive relationships with a primary carer from birth, but attachment requires a dyad in which an adult responds to a baby's emotional and physical needs and provides the optimum conditions for development. These conditions provide nurture and encourage the baby's overtures for a supportive relationship. Insecure attachment is exhibited by an inability to self-regulate; therefore, the accompanying conditions must change in order to promote agency and a sense of self.

Social learning through copying the role model of primary carers can be described as a key source of children's behaviour. Parenting programmes focus upon the promotion of positive behaviour by giving parents understanding of their negative responses and the impact upon the child's learning and development. Positive strategies can be implemented with optimum value if the parent's psychological resources are used to increase his or her capacity and ability to fulfil the parenting role. A parent's experience is founded upon his or her own childhood, in addition to parenting skills that accumulate through caring for several children in a family. A child's additional support needs can present a new experience and challenges to the parent's executive functioning as she learns to interpret and to respond the child's understanding of the world. Practitioners should support parents to use prior knowledge with confidence in addition to embracing learning opportunities and new parenting skills.

Environmental enrichment is a term that describes intervention in the form of stimulation and opportunities for development which are directly targeted to individual children or families. The ecological systems theory (Bronfenbrenner, 1979) portrays the potential of influences to impact upon the developing child by presentation in the form of concentric circles. The micro-system, meso-system, exo-system, and macro-system are composed of influences from different sources that can impact directly and indirectly upon the child's ability and capacity to progress. Although plasticity is regarded as being most relevant to the critical periods of learning in the earliest years, factors can continue to shape neural connections throughout a lifespan.

Toxic stress can affect the architecture of the brain, and this finding is significant to early intervention work and the necessity of supports by multi-agencies. I find that sources of stress are often described by parents as environmental and circumstantial, for example poor housing, poverty, and neighbourhood discrimination. Alleviation of these factors does not necessarily result in a reduction of toxic stress. Implicit memories which are based upon emotions can reproduce the stress reactions although the original source is minimised. Parents and grandparents will frequently, and emotively, recount historical instances of sexual abuse to service-providers and exhibit emotions from a childlike perspective.

It is challenging as a practitioner to respond with the optimum support as disclosures usually occur in unexpected circumstances. For example, within my workplace the cloakroom area is a regular discussion venue for parents to exhibit help-seeking behaviours to professionals (Broadhurst, 2003; Braun et al., 2006). Since the COVID-19 restrictions to building access have been in place, parents will frequently discuss issues in the carpark, which is the designated area for drop-off and pick-up between parent and service-provider (Scottish Government, 2020). Awareness of potential data confidentiality breaches can impose pressure on practitioners during such encounters in public spaces; however, parents' overtures should not be rejected. Ingenuity in communication media with families has been necessary during this uncertain period of the pandemic.

Therapeutic relationship

Hogg and Warne (2010) conducted a study on the responses to mental health by lay people. This term, as applied by the authors, referred to members of the public who did not have a professional designated role in the field of mental health. Participants in the research included a hairdresser, a parish priest, and a bar-worker. Responses from people in these roles to service-users, in a general public domain, had previously been described by Hochschild (1983) as emotional labour. This concept included management of people's emotions alongside tasks associated with a daily role or specific responsibilities. Differentiation can be made between the concepts of caring *for* someone, which encompasses physical, and environmental care, or caring *about* someone, which refers to a carer's responses to a service-user's needs and emotional reactions (Hogg & Warne, 2010).

The study by Hogg and Warne (2010) published interesting findings by highlighting the significant impact from lay people upon the mental health of a population. Skills of empathy, sensitive responding, and a non-judgemental attitude can accompany daily encounters between familiar and unfamiliar people and contribute effectively to good mental health in a community. Rogers (1990) had categorically stated that specialist knowledge, which is based upon professional training, is not required in the creation of a therapeutic relationship. The research by Rogers identified that relationships with friends can have therapeutic qualities which may be exhibited momentarily or arise periodically throughout relational interactions.

The research by Rogers (1990) also highlighted the longevity and consistency which could be achieved in a therapeutic relationship between a professional and client in a context of mental health. Rogers' six conditions are used as a framework for the creation and maintenance of therapeutic relationships and continue to influence guidance and practice today.

1   Two people in a psychological contact.
2   One person, a client in a state of incongruence.
3   The second person, a therapist in a state of congruence.
4   The therapist experiences unconditional positive regard for the client.
5   The therapist experiences empathic understanding of the client's frame of reference and communicates this to the client.
6   This communication is achieved to a minimal degree.

Rogers (1990) expressed that these six conditions require to exist over a period of time in order to inform constructive personality change in the client. One of Rogers' colleagues, Lyon (2014a, 2014b) summarised conditions on the characteristics of an effective teacher. Lyon identified one outcome as the trust that emerged within practice led by the six conditions. Tausch (2014) was another colleague of Rogers and Lyon, and his research findings indicated that non-genuineness created a relationship of mistrust. Demonstration of these conditions in practice do not simply affect each dyadic relationship but contribute to a positive atmosphere that permeates through a service. A practitioner who has knowledge, understanding, and capacity to use these interpersonal skills is extremely valuable to a service, particularly if his or her responsibilities encompass a leadership or supervisory role.

Lyon (2014a) and Rogers (1990) agreed that a challenge for the therapist was supporting the client to set and to achieve a goal of functioning positively. Lyon (2014a, 2014b) described the process of giving power to a developing person by nurturing his or her ability to operate independently from the therapist. It seems that power is knowledge and understanding in this context which leads to availability and extension of choices. This requires each person to recognise and to make choices that reflect his inner working model of beliefs, ideas, interests, and standards of living. A professional in early years care and education may have gained knowledge of mental-health issues through training, but comprehension and application of a skill set requires time and experience. However, every newly qualified or experienced early years practitioner can empower a parent, child, or colleague by generously sharing expertise, cooperating, collaborating, and nurturing the other person's capacity and ability.

Over the past thirty years, there have been several studies conducted that elucidate the characteristics of a professional and service-user relationship and reflect the six conditions of Rogers (1990). Smith (1992) conducted a study on the caring relationship within general nursing, and she clearly identifies the importance of role-modelling of the therapeutic alliance by a senior staff. The research indicated that the nursing team followed cues from their ward sister or charge nurse by using a therapeutic relationship to deliver care to patients. The team also commented on the benefit to each professional from the positive nurturing atmosphere which was created throughout the wards.

Stickley and Freshwater (2002) described love with healing potential as representation of the therapeutic relationship between nurse and patient.

These authors noted the challenge for nurses in creating a relationship of care and caring. This two-pronged relationship included delivering intervention within the parameters of disciplinary role and responsibilities in addition to responding to a patient's emotional well-being. Reference is made to Rogers (1990) and one of his core conditions for a therapeutic relationship: the counsellor experiences unconditional positive regard for the client. Nurses encounter patients who have a broad range of home circumstances, and it is essential that a non-judgemental professional approach is maintained at all times.

Early years practitioners and parents equate the delivery of care, education, and nurture with professional love (Whitters, 2019). This is not a replacement for parental love, which is unconditional between primary carer and child. Professional love is created for a purpose within the specific context of a service. This purpose broadly relates to holistic development of the child or parent which includes good mental health. The love projected from the practitioner to the family is unconditional on an emotional level, but it is formed within conditions that inherently create boundaries and recognisable parameters to the creation and maintenance of the relationship. Time, context, environment, and characteristics of each person are a few of the factors that define this type of love between service-provider and service-user. The human emotion of professional love encompasses a therapeutic connection between two human beings that portrays respect, and it promotes responsive care in a context of learning and development (Whitters, 2019). A highly valued and necessary skill is communicating belief in each person that he or she can achieve.

Emotional intelligence was investigated by McQueen (2004) in a literature review within a context of nursing studies. The use of emotional intelligence was identified as adoption of strategies to protect the mental health and well-being of professionals. Strategies included adequate supervision of general, and individual practice, in addition to periods of reflection and learning time. This author also promoted the use of emotional intelligence in negotiations within multidisciplinary teams, in the nursing context. Findings indicated the importance of emotional labour, but McQueen also warned about the potential for emotional burnout in a professional if the outlay was prolonged or intensive.

The pedagogical culture of any workplace has an important impact upon the delivery of a service, which inherently links to the well-being of employees and their capacity to use emotional labour with emotional intelligence. The service-provider and service-user relationship is a medium for communication, interaction, promotion of key issues, and transforming knowledge into understanding regardless of the context being health or care and education in the early years. Healing of a whole person takes place physically, emotionally, and socially within a therapeutic alliance. Professional love is demonstrated within a sensitive and responsive attitude towards an individual's emotional needs at a point of time, and it is accompanied by actions that promote development and minimisation of adversities. An early years worker practises in a role that encompasses interpersonal and intrapersonal aspects of care provision. Parents and children may gravitate towards practitioners, ancillary staff, or peers who demonstrate skills that match their areas of need. Parents may also choose to seek support from lay people due to freedom from conditions and expectations of these relationships.

Bowles and Jones (2005) discuss the concept of protection time in a context of mental-health nursing. These authors describe an inbuilt allocation of time within each shift which could be used to form a therapeutic relationship with a patient. Early years services are bound by adult–child ratios, but protected time can be gained through effective deployment of staffing at a local level. For example, the head of a service or senior practitioner may not be allocated within these ratios, or absences of children may result in fewer practitioners required to work directly with a group of children. In my experience, this protected time between parent and practitioner can also arise unexpectedly and can be capitalised upon. An example relates to the induction session in which a new child to the nursery is accompanied by his parent; therefore, he is not counted in the service adult–child ratios. Parents frequently use this first contact with a service to seek out emotional support. Information from a referring agent often provides the focal point of the meeting, and it acts as a catalyst for a parent to divulge his or her fears, anxieties, adversities, and to express emotional reactions. An induction session is conducive to a help-seeking context for a parent. The therapeutic alliance is a significant aspect of service-delivery, and protected time to support mental health needs should be given due consideration within health, education, and care services.

Parents may actively reject interaction with professionals or may not be aware of the route to accessing this support (Rogers & Pilgrim, 1997). In any service, child protection is paramount, and it is essential that the entire team, regardless of role, is trained in this area of work and takes responsibility to share information by following policies and procedures. Parents should always be aware that information is being shared, to whom, and the reason. The only caveat to withholding this communication from parents is the potential for a child to be harmed as a response to data-sharing between professionals in a child-protection context.

There are many mitigating factors to progress which are unpredictable, for example, chronic illness of parent or child or a diagnosis of a self-limiting illness. These barriers to change and development can create undue pressure on development of parenting skills. Holmes (2014) had promoted acceptance, courage, and adjustment to daily living as desirable outcomes for parents in these adverse contexts.

Parenting responses

Holmes (2014) reviewed parenting programmes from around the world and identified five common approaches within a context of early intervention.

1   Parent and child are supported alongside each other within a programme.
2   Child receives support within a programme.

3   Parent is the primary participant in a child-focused programme.
4   Parent is primary participant in a generic programme.
5   Parent and child are primary participants in an intervention programme.

Many services are adopting a therapeutic approach to behaviour management which has been re-termed as promotion of positive behaviour. The adult acknowledges the child's feelings and associated actions as a basis for promoting his sense of self and to guide him into replacing negative behaviours with positive. The young child is supported to recognise and to make positive choices that are proportionate to the social circumstances and cultural boundaries. The response by an adult is commonly termed "mind mindedness", which contributes to the child's maturation of the autobiographical self and the theory of mind.

The use of behaviour-management strategies by parents and professionals may affect the relationship on a temporary basis, but this cycle of rupture and repair is common. Children learn that relationships can be sustained despite these negative communications. Boundary-setting is a responsibility of a primary carer which supports socialisation, the child's comprehension of cause and effect, ownership of actions, and acceptance of consequences.

Adversities and poor mental health are not exclusively relevant to families who live in deprivation with outcomes of low attainment. Vaivre-Douret (2003) reported that development in children of extraordinary ability could be related to many high-level potentialities linked to functioning within the neuron networks. A property of cerebral functioning is plasticity, which provides opportunities for adaptation and regulation in response to influences. Findings from the study indicated that particular maturational developmental processing occurs in children who demonstrate higher ability than the chronological average. Plasticity in cerebral functioning is key to a child achieving his potential and actualising his desire for knowledge, but higher-than-average ability can also create vulnerability in a young child through a sense of frustration, isolation, and injustice. Vaivre-Douret concluded that high ability may coincide with neuropsychological or psychopathological disorders which are genetically based.

Genetic and environmental influences

Vaivre-Douret (2003) conducted research in the pre-birth and post-birth period. He identified that physiological development of the nervous and neuromuscular systems is affected by genetic and environmental factors, directly and indirectly. For example, an expectant mother may improve her diet during pregnancy and create a direct influence upon the foetus's development. This positive effect originates from an external source but creates an internal change. The mother's mental-health condition may deteriorate throughout the pregnancy and affect her well-being, which in turn has an indirect influence upon the foetus in-utero development.

Another factor to consider, in the context of an infant's development, is the creation of neural links at greater speed than the norm. Interactive processes which take place between genetic and environmental factors can modify the speed in development of nervous and neuromuscular systems within a child (Vaivre-Douret, 2011). A salient point is made by findings within the previous research of Vaivre-Douret (2003). This researcher noted that a child of high ability may rapidly acquire the solution to a problem but be reticent in exposing his skills to peers or adults. Findings indicated that this behaviour can be interpreted as emotional immaturity but actually represents hyper-maturity. This is due to the increased level and speed of information-processing capacity and analytical abilities. Normative responses of children with high ability may be demonstrated at an earlier age than peers and indicate greater intent and purpose within learning contexts. In accordance with this research, processes include attitudes and values placed upon educational attainment by primary carers that influence the child's engagement and involvement with learning.

Silverman (2016) described signs of ability as good memory, an early retention and use of a wide vocabulary, excessive physical activity, shorter sleep periods than the average child, sensitivity to the emotions of others, and a preference for playing with older peers. It is significant that these traits encompass intellectual, physical, and emotional development.

Unusual alertness is observed in some babies at birth and during forthcoming weeks and months. This characteristic is recognised as an indicator of high ability (Silverman, 2016). The baby will seek out eye contact with familiar caring adults and maintain this communication strategy for longer than expected of an infant. The baby will also seek out eye contact with unfamiliar adults in his proximal environment as an inherent response to a learning opportunity. He may conduct lengthy observations, and consideration of these circumstances, before engaging positively or seeking reassurance from a primary carer.

It is important to note that alertness in babies and children can also be observed in contexts of adversity. A baby who lives in a daily environment of potential danger, for example, parents with addictions, domestic violence, or abuse, may demonstrate vigilance. This human emotional reaction to fear is initially instinctive but develops into learned behaviour in accordance with home circumstances. It relates to personal safe-guarding strategies that can incur the baby demonstrating unusually focused and lengthy observations of his proximal environment. This knowledge equips the baby to determine a level of threat and to inform his subsequent actions.

Tronick and Beeghly (2011) highlight the negative effect upon the making of meaning if adversities are prolonged. These authors describe meaning-making as a transactional process in the lifespan which is supported through learning within a dyad, for example, mother–infant and practitioner–infant. The baby who is regarded as a developing system loses emotional stability, and he becomes vulnerable to effects of further threat if he experiences long-term toxic stress (Whitters, 2020).

Asmussen et al. (2020) advised that adversities may incur deprivation of intellectual stimulation. Overcoming this detrimental effect requires particular adaptation by a child. A further consequence of significant negative influences within childhood is highlighted as alteration of processing associated with threat, reward and memory which can be impactful upon social-emotional functioning. The result can be accumulative stress responses throughout the lifespan which originated from an initial childhood adversity. This research team suggested that resilience may be achieved through positive relationships with adults and peers. The study concludes by raising a question on whether resilience is an outcome of these secure attachments, or perhaps particular resilience characteristics of the child facilitate the creation of supportive relationships. It is always interesting when research presents a reader with a question to consider and to ponder – and potentially to investigate.

Motor development and physical prowess can be observed in some children at an earlier stage than the norm. The infant will rapidly recognise and respond to opportunities and actively seek out circumstances in which to practise his skills. In accordance with Vaivre-Douret (2011), sequencing of motor skill commences from fertilisation. Following birth, the order of sensorial and motor systems' development is cutaneous sensitivity, vestibular, gustatory, olfactory, auditory, and visual aspects. In a prior research study by Vaivre-Douret (2003), findings had indicated that children of high ability were observed to use their eyes and head in a noticeably active manner immediately after birth. The average newly born baby will be able to hold his head in axis for about two seconds, and after one month this motor skill will greatly increase. A baby with high ability can develop this skill more rapidly.

A focus on communication is common in the early years, and many young children seek out interaction between adults and books. This interest can stem from the close physical and emotional contact that arises when an adult and child share a book. Children of high ability often exhibit a keen interest in verbal and written communication and demonstrate an ability to link these two. Engaging with literature, without an adult's presence, can commence independently from an early stage of development. Recognition of letters can be retained more easily than peers, and the child may have an insatiable appetite for identifying familiar letters or words throughout his play environment within the home and community. Expressive and receptive language, including the use of grammar and tenses, are above average levels in accordance with age-group (Vaivre-Douret, 2003). First-time parents may not have an awareness that their child has high ability until the regular developmental checks are conducted by a health professional.

Alternatively, a child of high ability may be silent and demonstrate a tendency to learn by conducting lengthy observations, copying actions in situ, or applying extensive memory. The child's expressive language is displayed later than his peers. A child may exhibit the use of formed sentences with appropriate grammar and inflection, albeit the child is older than his peers and he has not demonstrated the babbling stage of communication or incremental effect of acquiring language over time.

Imaginative skills and motivation to use learning are shown by a strong desire to access further knowledge and understanding within tasks, supported activities, or free play. "A thirst for knowledge" is often expressed by parents or grandparents in describing a young child's avid responses to the world. These anecdotal comments by primary carers are upheld by research (Vaivre-Douret, 2003) in this field which identifies the constant searching for knowledge and understanding as a characteristic of some children. Learning through the senses, sight, hearing, smell, touch, and taste, is experienced with greater intensity than the average child, and the rich feedback of information can result in a vivid imagination which is accompanied by powerful emotional reaction. Heightened emotional reactions can be observed in children which depict their personal experience or portray a reaction and adoption of the emotions of others. This characteristic is founded on the child's capacity to experience empathy, and to understand the world from another person's perspective at a young age.

Personality and demeanour contribute to a child's reaction and interactions with learning processes. An infant may be extrovert and restless due to his quest for stimulation to fulfil his intellectual or physical needs. He may access adults as a source of knowledge and stimulation in his learning journey, but he can be attributed labels that actually describe the adult's inability to support the young child's needs: demanding, challenging, and non-compliant. If adults do not differentiate for the child's needs, then he may demonstrate unruly behaviour based upon rejection and his dissatisfaction. Research has linked behavioural disorders and disaffection with non-fulfilment of an infant's learning needs (Vaivre-Douret, 2003).

Alternatively, an infant may have a quiet, shy, or even introverted personality. He may use personal strategies to fulfil his needs by himself. For example, I have often observed a young child presenting increasingly difficult challenges to himself in play: problem-solving, remembering vast amounts of information, and calculating numerical goals with or without the use of external prompts. External prompts are accessed in accordance with the child's preferences in using one or more of his five senses: visual prompts through recording the information in writing or electronically, auditory prompts through reciting information or substituting tapping for counting internally. A quiet child will often accelerate his own learning, or use enrichment by exploring topics in depth, and ultimately a multitude of sources of information become his teachers. Reciprocal interaction emerges between the child and his preferred media of knowledge, as opposed to interaction within a carer or peer relationship. Intellectual stimulus abounds but emotional and social stimuli are depleted.

Box 3.3 Example from practice

The context was an orange and green double-decker bus in Glasgow city centre, the 34 bus to the Southside. It was seven o'clock in the morning, and I was travelling to work alongside a motley assortment of fellow employees: office workers who were neat and tidy, keen to embrace the daily tasks, students in jeans and college sweatshirts with large, ubiquitous bags of knowledge slung across their shoulders, and night-shift staff who were tired and jaded, ready to go home and sleep during daylight hours. As a childcare worker, I notice children and parents in every context, and my interest was alerted as a young mother climbed aboard with a buggy.

The time was autumn of 2020 as the COVID-19 pandemic continued to encompass our world. My fellow travellers wore face-coverings, and we were separated carefully by definitive signs on each seat that welcomed or rejected a potential user. We sat quietly, socially distanced, behind, and diagonally, COVID-safe. This vantage point was useful as I could see the buggy and occupant clearly. A little girl with masses of dark curls peeked around her rain cover. I considered her age to be 12 months.

I smiled broadly as a generic introduction to any young child; however, masks only reveal smiling eyes, and the little girl was too young to interpret my overture. She frowned and dipped her head back inside the security of her buggy hood. Disappointed, I glanced out of the dark window and could only see reflections of streetlights shining against the still water of the river Clyde. The bus moved smoothly across the bridge, and I returned my gaze to the bright interior. The scenario had developed. The young mother had given her child an identity badge. I recognised the health-service colours on this badge, and I wondered about the mother's role.

The child was fascinated by this new toy, and it was obvious that her involvement and well-being were high. I noticed that the little girl had mastered the skill of observation and planning. She used two hands, liberating ten fine motor tools as her fingers felt the webbing on the lanyard. Strangely, I found myself touching the lanyard of my own identification badge, which was hidden from view and tucked inside my winter jacket. For a few moments, I thought about the processes of learning, applicable to all human beings, young and old. I had followed a basic learning principle of copying by emulating this little girl's movements.

The fastening on a lanyard requires opposing forces to release it, although professionals in public-health fields are usually issued with sophisticated versions with a quick safety release in case of assault by a client, but the hard sharp pull required in this context was beyond the capability of a 12-month-old learner.

The girl leant forward, and I had a front-seat row to view the drama. She rapidly found the plastic clip and momentarily put it into her mouth. I watched the scene unfolding, and I was fascinated by the child's competent use of her five senses within this exploratory task. Two hands worked together, first attempt then one failure, two attempts then success, and the two ends of the lanyard sprang apart. The child rubbed her curls back and forward against the buggy in celebration and smiled to herself. Goal achieved!

Common daily scenes depict the ability and capacity of a child at a point in time. The motor and coordination skills that this child applied were developed in situ, and the achievement of the planned outcome demonstrated motivation to learn within the task.

Internal and external asynchrony

Silverman (2016) described higher-than-average ability as atypical development, and she highlights aspects of internal and external asynchrony.

- **Internal asynchrony** relates to different rates of growth in the child's physical, intellectual, and emotional development compared to the norm for his or her age group.
- **External asynchrony** can occur during the child's interactions with a learning environment as compared to the norm. The child's interpretation and reactions to objects and circumstances usually differ from the peer group and expectations of adults.

Differentiation and integration

Learning is a sensory, emotional, and intellectual experience in which the sense of self can be affirmed or changed. Csikszentmihalyi (1990) describes flow theory as a process in which the understanding of a sense of self increases, and extends, by the use of two psychological processes. He identifies these processes as differentiation and integration.

Differentiation occurs as the person gains an increase in skill and capacity, and application of knowledge is greater. **Integration** is achieved as thoughts and emotions are focused upon the same goal and result in a deeper level of understanding. Findings by Csikszentmihalyi (1990) indicated that differentiation emphasises *individuality* whereas integration can support identification and *connection with others* who demonstrate a similar interpretation and comprehension of a learning environment.

Four steps are identified by Csikszentmihalyi (1990) in the achievement of flow during processes of learning, and the term **autotelic self** indicates an overarching sense of purpose as experienced by the individual. As I consider these steps, I am reminded of my 12-month-old fellow passenger on the number 34 bus in Glasgow.

1 Setting goals.
2 Involvement in an activity.
3 Focused attention.
4 High level of intellectual involvement and emotional well-being in current experience.

Task commitment is closely associated with motivation to seek out learning opportunities. McCoach and Flake (2018) describe motivation as domain-

and task-specific. The alignment or non-alignment between the factors of domain and task represents flow theory and directly affects motivation.

Flow theory

Flow theory refers to the influences from two variables upon a child's experiences.

1   Situational features are the challenges or facilitators that an activity presents to the child from the proximal environment. The parent or practitioner has a direct impact upon this influence.
2   Personal characteristics are the child's own skill set which encompasses personality, emotions, and reaction to the world.

Flow theory is a subjective experience in which a young learner feels alert, competent, fulfilled, and also motivated to remain on his continuum of learning and achievement. Csikszentmihalyi (1990) spent many years researching concepts associated with optimal experience, and he identified six characteristics of flow theory described from an infant's internal perspective:

1   He merges actions and awareness. Awareness is relative to an infant's stage of a sense of self.
2   He is fully concentrating on the present situation.
3   He explores without being self-consciousness.
4   His body language expresses an expectation of success.
5   He senses that time is speeding up or slowing down during the interaction.
6   He has a desire to engage in the activity for the experience of joy, termed autotelic motivation.

It is widely accepted that there are three ways in which knowledge is acquired in the early years. The first approach is an infant observing and copying in situ. For example, if an adult sticks out his tongue in close proximity to a 6-week-old baby, then he will copy the action as long as the prompt remains visible. The second approach entails an infant observing and reproducing an action from memory in the short term. For example, if an adult demonstrates a practical instruction of putting one brick on top of another before taking the bricks apart and creating a learning space, then the infant will attempt to reproduce these actions. The young infant may require reminders of the actions required to build the tower of bricks if the visual prompt is no longer available. The final approach is an infant internalising instructions and applying knowledge, or collaborative learning with peers and adults in a variety of contexts, and time frames. For example, if an infant attempts to touch a specific hot surface, the carer will firmly say "No" and actively stop the child's hand from completing this action. On subsequent occasions, the adult will simply say "No" without the practical prompt, and an infant will internalise representation of this word as cause and effect in the context of the aforementioned hot surface. Over time, an infant will acquire the ability to extrapolate actions and meaning associated with the word "No" to other similar contexts.

Vygotsky (1978) studied the social nature of learning throughout his career, and he believed that co-constructivism provided the optimum context in which potential could be achieved; however, one child may have greater control over environmental change and internal representation than another. An increase in intrinsic motivation can serve to minimise distractions from external events or adversities which can be observed in the performance of some infants. These infants have greater independence and less reliance on the environment as a prompt for learning. The children require fewer stimuli from the environment than their peers in order to achieve internal representation of consciousness in a context of knowledge and understanding. Parents and practitioners have often commented to me in reference to an independent young child, "He can find learning opportunities in any situation!"

Alternatively, Csikszentmihalyi (1990) found that greater dependency on the external environment is required by some individuals to create a representation of reality. This knowledge of approaches to learning directly informs practice, and it underlines the importance of planning and of setting a playroom for infants and young children at different stages of development. Every practitioner develops skill in presenting choices to children at their developmental levels. It is always effective practice to have supplementary items prepared and ready to offer learners who rapidly achieve their goals in addition to learners who benefit from repetitive interactions with artefacts relating to lower levels of thinking.

Anxiety and boredom were identified by Csikszentmihalyi (1990) as two main impediments to enjoyment in life. Anxiety can occur if challenges are perceived as unachievable, and, conversely, boredom can arise if a child perceives his abilities as greater than the opportunities that are presented in a particular environment. Young children may not have an awareness of the reason for feeling boredom but exhibit unruly behaviour as a response to lack of stimulation from minimal learning experiences, or restrictive boundaries. The adult should seek to understand this medium of communication and to interpret the infant or child's behaviour. At times, I have heard carers comment, "There's no reason for this disruptive behaviour", in reference to unruly actions and aggressive tendencies. Anxiety or boredom often underlie these behavioural communications by a child. Challenging cognitive tasks or introducing new physical activities are useful responses. It is not always possible for workers to leave a playroom in order to bring new artefacts into the play arena, but ingenuity and enthusiasm from a team can support reconfiguration of resources to stimulate a child. Involving children in creating a new venture can channel emotions associated with anxiety or boredom towards emotions linked to achievement of a new task. Actions can support self-regulation as a child reinterprets his learning environment.

Zhou and Brown (2015) explored three approaches to changing behaviour which are applicable to all children within the earliest years of childhood: cueing, shaping, and modelling. Cueing is the use of verbal or non-verbal prompts that link specific behaviour to circumstances. Cueing is most effective if used to pre-empt negative behaviours by promotion of a positive change model rather than a response to a child's unsociable actions.

A child's responses can also be shaped by practical scaffolding or verbal interaction. Shaping entails an educator using strategies to incrementally support a child to change his behaviour. All the steps may be explained to the child at the outset of a task and linked to expectations and outcomes. The child gains awareness of changing his behaviour. Alternatively, the change process can be determined by an adult introducing each small step in context. The child may not have an awareness that his behaviour is changing through these subliminal accumulative steps. This lack of awareness can result in a child positively embracing a situation of change. If a child perceives that he is losing control of his environment, then he may rebel against the change through fear and anxiety associated with an unfamiliar situation.

Modelling is often described as role-modelling within a service in which an adult or peer actively demonstrates expectations of behaviour to a child throughout the generic context. Zhou and Brown (2015) make the important point that modelling can lead to diversion from the original source of learning. For example, a child can produce unique patterns of behaviour as he attempts to replicate the adult's actions. The use of child-led pedagogy has minimised the educator's focus upon predetermined goals and subsequently liberated children to demonstrate imaginative and creative skills.

Motivation

The research by Gottfried et al. (1994) referred to intrinsic motivation which was linked to the content of a task, a child's personal interests, and the experience of pleasure in intellectual attainment. The achievement of intellectual goals is experienced internally but may be rewarded externally by teachers or parents which can lead to dependency on external recognition. This study by Gottfried and his research team had focused upon a child's internal reward system and his motivation to seek out higher levels of understanding. Links were made between intrinsic motivation, giftedness, and pleasure which were associated with cognitive processing. Findings indicated that family circumstances, resources, and social status in a community had positive impact upon cognitive development; however, the study concluded that familial influences can also hinder or prevent the realisation of genetic potential.

Twenty-five years later, the same researcher, Gottfried (2019), collected data on adolescents' perceptions of their parents' support during young formative years. The adolescent participants expressed that task-intrinsic approaches by their parents were more effective than task-extrinsic. Findings indicated that a parent's affirmation of the child's internal emotional experience, and the child's recognition of his goal, supported learning processes.

The study by Kreppner (2001) had also noted particular responses in relation to mothers of children who had high ability. These mothers adapted their interactions and information-sharing with their children in accordance with developing cognitive skills. Additionally, Kreppner found that mothers of children who had lower abilities tended to interrupt the child's play and did not use instructions which reflected his maturation and changing abilities. This approach restricted the child's opportunities to access learning experiences and to broaden his understanding of the world.

If children gain pleasure and fulfilment during cognitive processing, then they will develop tendencies to engage with activities and pursuits which further these outcomes.

- Intrinsic value represents the child's apportioning of worth upon a task relative to his interests and personality.
- Attainment value has relevance to the child's own goals and his sense of self.
- Utility value impacts upon present or future goals and applications (McCoach & Flake, 2018).

Extrinsic motivation is instrumental due to dependency on an external reward. This reward may be tangible as a sticker or toy which is given to the child, or perhaps emotionally based in the form of praise, or socially based in the form of acceptance by a peer group, or, finally, culturally based integration within a family group. These outcomes are apportioned value by the child, and he may actively seek out specific rewards through his behaviour. Rewards incite the creation of behavioural patterns within daily interactions and incorporate expectations of the child and caregiver.

Intervention

Stern (2018) reviewed the purpose and effect of interventions which are delivered in a context of therapeutic support. He described therapeutic intervention as building upon a relationship of trust between parent and therapist. This foundation creates a medium for effective communication and the parent's belief and acceptance in the therapist's input, which increases the value of the intervention. Stern also commented that many interventions encompass a rationale of a strengths-based approach that focuses upon a parent's current skill set instead of areas for development. This approach was described by Stern as superficial interventions of support as opposed to therapies.

Stern (2018) advocated therapies that promote understanding and ultimately acceptance of past events. One strategy is giving a parent knowledge and a rationale for using sensitive responding between adult and child. For example, child–parent psychotherapy assists a family in exposing emotions and reactions to trauma and gaining resilience to negative impact. Contextualising the negative experiences, in addition to comprehending and accepting the accompanying emotions, can support a parent's ability to change and develop. Over time, parents can be supported to reflect upon experiences that change their perceptions of the parenting role and responsibilities. A therapeutic alliance between therapist and parent can contribute to the parent's capacity to show empathy towards a child. The therapist's unconditional positive regard is a key factor in this process in which the parent's inner working model is reconfigured, leading to a change in perceptions, actions, and reactions.

The therapist in child–parent psychotherapy guides these complex processes by nurturing links between internal beliefs and external behaviours. The term "port of entry" applied by Lieberman et al. (2019) refers to the use of spontaneous behaviour, interactions, and free play within the intervention session to capitalise upon potential for change in parent and child. Personalities, temperament, and identified clinical issues are often determining factors in the therapist prioritising a port of entry. Blechman (2016) particularly highlighted the transition period in which a parent commences the process of change. During this time, the parent learns to express problems in an abstract manner and gradually identifies solutions and applies concrete actions within the circumstances of daily living. Blechman believed that solutions encompassed overt words and actions, in addition to covert thoughts and feelings of the individual.

Lieberman et al. (2019) also reviewed family intervention therapy, which specifically targets areas of change for parents, and children from birth to five years, by focusing upon negative aspects of family life. Findings indicate that trauma-informed treatment promotes knowledge and understanding that supports reconfiguration of the parent's and child's inner working models. Examples of areas for change were given by the researchers as unsafe environmental conditions, mental-health issues that have an adverse impact upon the parent–child relationship, and maladaptive internal and external parent or child behaviours. Internal behaviour can include difficulty in recognising and expressing emotions, which can lead to social withdrawal. Reaction to adversities may be demonstrated externally through aggression and a desire for excessive control of situations.

The rationale of child–parent psychotherapy is presented by the therapist during play sessions with parent and child. A link between parent's and child's actions and reactions is explored, and the caregiver is supported to identify negative and ameliorative factors. These factors may be current or based upon historical experiences. The child and parent learn to put their trauma experiences into context and to differentiate between remembering and reliving the events and emotions. The therapist promotes parent and child engagement with developmental goals and guides the parent to shape a future positive family life.

Research indicates that the therapeutic alliance is strengthened by the skill of each therapist in facilitating discussion of traumatic events. This positive context encompasses change, development, and an increase in mental well-being of child, parent, and extended family (Lieberman et al., 2019). The context of an intervention therapy is essential to give the parent and child a means of controlling the emotional impact of trauma within a safe environment. Families learn to rationalise and to compartmentalise the adversities within their own time frames. The family members also learn how to create a new framework for daily living in which negativity is replaced with positivity and hope for a better future.

I work in a care setting that implements therapeutic pedagogy throughout all activities and places significance on nurturing practitioner–parent, practitioner–child, and parent–child relationships. Families attend the service to access a nursery placement in addition to parenting support. Referring agents, for example, social work, addictions, and health professionals, identify the adversities and the impact upon each member of a family. Formal interventions are promoted that support this process of change and development. However, parents also choose to share trauma experiences informally at times which are opportune to their emotions, well-being, and understanding of specific practitioner–parent relationships. These interactions often occur outwith an allocated intervention session, and it is important that the practitioner is equipped to respond sensitively within this moment of personal disclosure by a parent. In recent years, training in adverse childhood experiences, neural processes, and trauma-informed practice have become key core components of continuous professional development for registered practitioners.

Play as therapy

Play that is based upon experiences of trauma provides rich and valid opportunities to create narratives that respond to emotional issues in a safe and protected environment. The review by Lieberman et al. (2019) also promoted an ongoing narrative by the therapist as an effective strategy to alter perceptions and interpretation of actions. The play is tracked by the therapist throughout a session. This specific use of words to express actions and accompanying emotions has great value in increasing understanding of parent and child. The therapist encourages the parent to demonstrate nurture and love through physical contact with a child. I have found that this context can be challenging for some parents. Role-modelling by a practitioner is a useful approach to experiential learning for a parent. In every interaction between adults and children, there are multiple opportunities to demonstrate respect, care, and love.

In the mid-1960s, a husband-and-wife team of researchers created the filial therapy model in which recognition is given to parents' use of play-therapy principles and skills within adult–child interactive play sessions (Guerney, 1964). This model responded to the mental-health needs of young children and continues to be implemented today. Adaptation includes the use of a trained practitioner in the role of facilitator, for example, a key worker within an early years service (Morrison & Helker, 2010). The therapeutic skills can be extrapolated beyond the intervention and applied by the facilitator within any other environment in which interaction occurs between adult and child (Post, 2010). This transitional feature of child–teacher relationship training is supportive for the child's transference of self-belief, emotional literacy, and self-regulation within common daily contexts.

Child-centred play therapy is another effective intervention that targets the mental health of a child and parent (Baggerly, 2010). The child participates in sessions of interactive play, supported by his parent or trained facilitator. The conceptual toys stimulate the child's exploration and increased understanding of his emotions in relation to trauma. The adult reflects the child's non-verbal behaviour, emotions, ability, and capacity to overcome challenges. The rationale of this intervention stems from the belief in the child's increasing capacity to gain an understanding of self and to regulate his emotions and actions. Ray and Edwards (2010) promoted the role of adult as facilitating an environment of permissiveness and freedom to understand and to make choices. The optimum outcome is the child's transference of this learning to environments out-with the therapeutic context.

Fall (2010) describes self-efficacy as belief in oneself. It is this belief that can create reparation links between adversities and a positive fulfilling life. The reparation element is founded upon an increase in knowledge, understanding, and resilience, in addition to appointing value and respect to oneself. This belief is necessary for an individual to create internal change and the confidence to express these changes externally.

Nurturing this belief is a key aspect of trauma-informed practice. Self-belief can increase dramatically within multiple contexts: formal and informal intervention and daily living experiences. Short interactions between an attachment figure and a child can engender self-belief, and the output from an interaction does not rely upon a specific timescale. Play therapy reinforces strengths but acknowledges weaknesses. Tracking phrases contribute to the child's creation of a trauma and a resilience narrative. Facilitator responses are built upon principles of acceptance and change.

- Acknowledge the child's actions and accompanying emotion.
- Communicate the social boundary.
- Target an alternative action within the session context which responds to the child's need and emotion at this point of time.

Bandura (1997) had identified the formation of self-efficacy judgements based upon the blending of four influences: mastery experiences, social experiences, social influences, and physiological responses. Tyndall-Lind (2010) conducted research on shared play-therapy sessions with siblings who had experienced domestic violence in their home environment. The study explored these influences in relation to each child. Findings indicated that the play flow was fluid throughout the sessions, and there was evidence of secure attachment between the children. The sibling relationships, and play-therapy context, provided appropriate conditions for the children to experience, and to practise, different behaviours with one another. Participants were also able to access conceptual toys in this safe, predictable setting. The study applied the term "therapeutic partners" to the brothers' and sisters' relationships.

Animals are also known to represent secure attachment to children in this context of therapeutic partners. Research indicates that physical contact with a pet animal triggers a release of neuropeptides that results in the child experiencing a feeling of security and comfort. Findings from a research study highlighted positive effects from animal relationships upon children who had been emotionally and socially abused (Doyle & Timms, 2014).

Stern (2018) regarded the child's development as impacting greatly on repeat or extended intervention. This researcher explained that each session supports a parent to make changes to his parenting responses, but week four of a therapy will be delivering intervention to a child who has developed since week one. An initial intervention, repeat interventions, and extended sessions should recognise that the child and parent have a continuously evolving foundation of knowledge and understanding.

During video feedback sessions, I have observed that parents can easily identify their negative parenting interactions or lack of reaction to the child's overtures. However, with encouragement, the parents can also identify positive skills and reconfigure their understanding of each scenario by making suggestions for change. The child adapts alongside the parent, and positive effect can occur quickly. The reconfigured approach is presented to the child in the context of developmental changes which are occurring continuously; therefore, the parent needs be motivated and alert to embracing and adapting to change as it occurs. Empowerment of primary carers is a key factor in promoting interventions with longevity of outcomes.

In my experience, many parents request extra sessions of parenting support. Stern (2018) suggested that parents gain value from the therapeutic relationship in addition to the practical strategies. Memory of the positive relationship, and the accompanying belief that the therapist demonstrates to a parent, can maintain the momentum of an intervention after completion. A therapeutic relationship between therapist, or early years practitioner and parent, will eventually come to an end as the child moves between age-appropriate services.

Fatigue

Professional fatigue is a mental-health issue that has come to the fore in recent years, and this condition has been highlighted repeatedly by the media during the current COVID-19 pandemic. However, stress can also be stimulating and lead to professionals achieving optimum performance within their disciplines, as described by Ulrich-Lai and Herman (2009). These authors identified that stress may represent positive stimuli and the physiological effect is similar to that of stress that induces negative effects. The research revealed that delight/elation and fear/terror produced similar biological reactions.

Additionally, findings indicated that reward behaviours reduced stress responses by creating physiological *and* psychological change.

It is well known that healthy eating and regular exercise impact positively upon long-term stress. During the lockdown periods of 2020 and 2021, populations throughout many countries were allocated short daily exercise times outside as a means to improve mental health. There was also a noticeable increase in the public's engagement with physical activity via indoor media across all age groups. Throughout our lifespans, the hippocampus generates neurons. Exercise is linked to this process of neurogenesis (Erikkson et al., 1998) by generating neurotrophic proteins that are responsible for growth, maintenance, and survival of neurons. It may be the case that the increase in society's focus upon exercise and well-being will continue after the effects of the pandemic have reduced.

References

Asmussen, K., Fischer, F., Drayton, E., & McBride, T. (2020). Adverse childhood experiences: What we know, what we don't know, and what should happen next. https://members.childlink.co.uk/document/adverse-childhood-experiences-what-we-know-what-we-don%E2%80%99t-know-and-what-should-happen-next?page=3.

Baggerly, J. N. (2010). Preface. In J. N. Baggerly, D. C. Ray, & S. C. Bratton (Eds.), *Child-centred play therapy research: The evidence base for effective practice* (pp. xiii–xviii). Hoboken, NJ: John Wiley.

Bandura, A. (1997). *Self-efficacy: The exercise of control.* New York: Freeman.

Belsky, J. (1984). The determinants of parenting: A process model. https://www.idoc.pub/documents/belsky-1984-determinants-of-parentinga-process-modelpdf-pqn8jpw23141.

Blechman, E. A. (2016). Effective communication: Enabling multi-problem families to change. In P. A. Cowan & M. Hetherington (Eds.), *Family Transitions* (pp. 219–244). Abingdon and New York: Routledge.

Bowles, N., & Jones, A. (2005). Whole systems working and acute inpatient psychiatry: An exploratory study. *Journal of Psychiatric and Mental Health Nursing* 12 (*3*), 283–289. https://www.onlinelibrary.wiley.com/doi/abs/10.1111/j.1365-2850.2005.00834.x.

Bratton, S. C., Landreth, G. L., Kellam, T., & Blackard, S. R. (2006). *Child/parent participation therapy treatment manual.* Abingdon and New York: Routledge.

Braun, D., Davis, H., & Mansfield, P. (2006). *How helping works: Towards a shared model of process.* London: Centre for Parent and Child Support.

Broadhurst, K. (2003). Engaging parents and carers with family support services: What can be learned from research on help-seeking? *Journal of Child and Family Social Work*, 10. http://onlinelibrary.wiley.com/doi/10.1046/j.1365-2206.2003.00289.x/abstract.

Bronfenbrenner, U. (1979). *The ecology of human development*, 2nd edition. Cambridge, MA: Harvard University Press.

Csikszentmihalyi, M. (1990). *Flow: The psychology of optimal experience.* New York: HarperCollins.

Department for Education and Skills. (2004). *The effective provision of pre-school education (EPPE) project: The final report.* Nottingham: Institute of Education.

Doyle, C., & Timms, C. (2014). *Child neglect and emotional abuse: Understanding, assessment and response.* London: Sage.

Erikkson, P. S., Perfilieva, E., Bjork-Eriksson, T., Alborn, A. M., Nordborg, C., Peterson, D. A., & Gage, F. H. (1998). Neurogenesis in the adult human hippocampus. *Nature Medicine, 4(11),* 1313–1317.

Fall, M. (2010). Increased self-efficacy: One reason for play therapy success. In J. N. Baggerly, D. C. Ray, & S. C. Bratton (Eds.), *Child-centred play therapy research: The evidence base for effective practice* (pp. 37–51). Hoboken, NJ: John Wiley & Sons.

Gottfried, A. E. (2019). Academic intrinsic motivation: theory, assessment, and longitudinal research. Journal of advances in motivation science, (6), 2019, 71–109, https://www.sciencedirect.com/science/article/abs/pii/S221509191830021X

Gottfried, A. E., Fleming, J. S., & Gottfried, A. W. (1994). Role of parental motivational practices in children's academic intrinsic motivation and achievement. *Journal of Educational Psychology, 86(1),* 1040113. https://fosteringintrinsicmotivation. weebly.com/uploads/2/5/0/3/25031030/role_of_parental_motivational_practices.pdf.

Guerney, B. G. (1964). Filial therapy: Description and rationale. *Journal of Consulting Psychology, 28(4),* 304–310. https://doi.org/10.1037/h0041340.

Hochschild, A. (1983). *The managed heart: Commercialisation of human feeling.* Berkeley, CA: University of California Press.

Hogg, C., & Warne, T. (2010). Ordinary people, extraordinary voices: The emotional labour of lay people caring for and about people with a mental health problem. *International Journal of Mental Health Nursing,* 19, 297–306.

Holmes, J. (2014). Where the child is the concern, working therapeutically with parents. In P. Holmes & S. Farnfield (Eds.), *The Routledge handbook of attachment: Implications and interventions* (pp. 53–64). Hove: Routledge.

Kreppner, K. (2001). Infant education. *International Encyclopedia of the Social and Behavioural Sciences,* 7414–7419. https://www.sciencedirect.com/science/article/pii/B0080430767023809.

Lieberman, A. F., Dimmler, M. H., & Ippen, C. M. G. (2019). Child–parent psychotherapy: A trauma-informed treatment for young children and their caregivers. In C. H. Zeanah (Ed.), *Handbook of infant mental health,* 4th edition (pp. 485–499). New York: The Guilford Press.

Lyon, H. (2014a). Educating the gifted and talented: Freedom to reach your potential. In C. R. Rogers, H. C. Lyon, & R. Tausch (Eds.), *On becoming an effective teacher: Person-centred teaching, psychology, philosophy, and dialogues with Carl R. Rogers and Harold Lyon* (pp. 47–57). Abingdon: Routledge.

Lyon, H. (2014b). Person-centred management and leadership. In C. R. Rogers, H. C. Lyon, & R. Tausch (Eds.), *On becoming an effective teacher: Person-centred teaching, psychology, philosophy, and dialogues with Carl R. Rogers and Harold Lyon* (pp. 95–103). Abingdon: Routledge.

McCoach, D. B., & Flake, J. K. (2018). The role of motivation. In S. I. Pfeiffer (Ed.), *APA handbook of giftedness and talent* (pp. 201–213). Washington, DC: American Psychological Association.

McQueen, A. (2004). Emotional intelligence in nursing work. *Journal of Advanced Nursing, 47(1),* 101–108. https://www.onlinelibrary.wiley.com/doi/abs/10.1111/j.1365-2648.2004.03069.x.

Montessori, M. (1964). *The Montessori method.* New York: Schocken Books. First published 1912.

Morrison, M. O., & Helker, W. P. (2010). An early mental health intervention for disadvantaged preschool children. In J. N. Baggerly, D. C. Ray, & S. C. Bratton (Eds.), *Child-centred play therapy research: The evidence base for effective practice* (pp. 427–447). Hoboken, NJ: John Wiley & Sons.

Panksepp, J. (1998). *Affective neuroscience: The foundations of human and animal emotions*. Oxford: Oxford University Press.

Plutchik, R. (1980). A general psycho-evolutionary theory of emotion. In R. Plutchik & H. Kellerman (Eds.), *Emotion: Theory, Research, and Experience* (pp. 3–33). New York: Academic Press.

Post, P. (2010). Child-centred kinder training for teachers of preschool children deemed at risk. In J. N. Baggerly, D. C. Ray, & S. C. Bratton (Eds.), *Child-centred play therapy research: The evidence base for effective practice* (pp. 409–427). Hoboken, NJ: John Wiley & Sons.

Ray, D. C., & Edwards, N. A. (2010). Play therapy effect on relationship stress. In J. N. Baggerly, D. C. Ray, & S. C. Bratton (Eds.), *Child-centred play therapy research: The evidence base for effective practice* (pp. 105–125). Hoboken, NJ: John Wiley & Sons.

Rogers, A., & Pilgrim, D. (1997). The contribution of lay knowledge to the understanding and promotion of mental health. *Journal of Mental Health*, 6(*1*). 23–35.

Rogers, C. (1990). Theory and research. In H. Kirschenbaum & V. L. Henderson (Eds.), *The Carl Rogers reader*, London: Constable.

Scottish Government. (2020). Early learning and childcare COVID-19 Update, No. 3–9, June. https://www.gov.scot/publications/coronavirus-covid-19-early-learning-childcare-services.

Scottish Government & NHS Scotland. (2021). Trauma-informed practice: A toolkit for Scotland. https://www.gov.scot/publications/trauma-informed-practice-toolkit-scotland.

Silverman, L. (2016). Early signs of giftedness. https://www.gifteddevelopment.com.

Siraj-Blatchford, I., Sylva, K., Taggart, B., Melhuish, E., Sammons, P., & Elliot, K. (2003). *The effective provision of pre-school education (EPPE) project (1997–2003)*. Nottingham: Department for Education and Skills.

Smith, P. (1992). *The emotional labour of nursing*. London: Macmillan.

Sroufe, A., Duggal, S., Weinfield, N., & Carlson, E. (2000). *Relationships, development, and psychopathology: Handbook of developmental psychology*, 2nd edition. New York: Kluwer Academic/Plenum Publishers.

Stern, D. N. (1998). *The interpersonal world of the infant*. London: H. Karnac.

Stern, D. N. (2018). *The motherhood constellation: A unified view of parent–infant psychotherapy*. Abingdon and New York: Routledge.

Stickley, T., & Freshwater, D. (2002). The art of loving and the therapeutic relationship. *Nursing Inquiry*, 9(4), 250–256.

Tausch, R. (2014). Research in Germany on person-centred methods: Teutonic thoroughness. In C. R. Rogers, H. C. Lyon, & R. Tausch (Eds.), *On becoming an effective teacher: Person-centred teaching, psychology, philosophy, and dialogues with Carl R. Rogers and Harold Lyon* (pp. 114–133). Abingdon and New York: Routledge.

Trevarthen, C., & Aitken, K. J. (2001). Infant intersubjectivity: Research, theory, and clinical applications. *Journal of Child Psychology and Psychiatry*, 42(1), 3–48.

Tronick, E., & Beeghly, M. (2011). Infants' meaning-making and the development of mental health problems. *American Psychologist*, 66(2), 107–109.

Tyndall-Lind, A. (2010). Intensive sibling group play therapy with child witnesses of domestic violence. In J. N. Baggerly, D. C. Ray, & S. C. Bratton (Eds.), *Child-centred play therapy research: The evidence base for effective practice.* Hoboken, NJ: John Wiley & Sons.

Ulrich-Lai, Y. M., & Herman, J. P. (2009). Neural regulation of endocrine and autonomic stress responses. *Nature Review: Neuroscience* 10, 397–409.

Vaivre-Douret, L. (2003). Early developmental characteristics in children with a high level of potential. *Journal français de psychiatrie* 1, 1–3. https://www.cairn-int.info/journal-journal-francais-de-psychiatrie-2003-1-page-I.htm.

Vaivre-Douret, L. (2011). Developmental and cognitive characteristics of "high-level potentialities" (highly gifted) children. *International Journal of Paediatrics, 420297.* https://www.researchgate.net/publication/51697095_Developmental_and_Cognitive_Characteristics_of_High-Level_Potentialities_Highly_Gifted_Children.

Vygotsky, L. S. (1978). *Mind in society: Development of higher psychological processes.* Cambridge, MA: Harvard University Press.

Whitters, H. G. (2018). *Family learning to inclusion in the early years.* Abingdon and New York: Routledge.

Whitters, H. G. (2019). Nurture … or is it love? EECERA: European Early Years Childcare and Education Research Association. https://www.eecera.org/gen/guest-post-nurture-or-love.

Whitters, H. G. (2020). *Adverse childhood experiences, attachment, and the early years learning environment.* Abingdon and New York: Routledge.

Zhou, M., & Brown, D. (2015). *Educational learning theories*, 2nd edition, Education Open Textbooks, 1. https://oer.galileo.usg.edu/education-textbooks/1.

4 Learning and adversities

Chapter 4 presents the infant and adult mind as a complex system that encompasses many layers and potential connections (Siegel, 2003). Mental health is described as a self-organising process that supports an individual to achieve maximum complexity by use of differentiation and integration. Uneven adaptation can occur as the mentalising resources are split between the external world and influences of others and the internal world of the individual and comprehension of his sense of self (Fonagy, 1999).

Multi-modal approaches are indicated which target different learning styles of families and can respond sensitively to increasing capacity and ability as time progresses. Examples of experiences throughout play environments are linked to activation of the child's genes. The result is protein production, which changes the architecture of the brain as new synapses form. Recent findings of Boyce et al. (2021) referred to individual susceptibility to adversity and links between unsupportive parenting and increased inflammatory reactions throughout the lifespan. Knowledge of the destructive properties of cortisol is used to inform the rationale for strategic planning and intervention (National Scientific Council on the Developing Child, 2006).

Adverse childhood experiences

Infants learn through interaction with the world, which creates an inner framework of reference to support understanding and inform actions. These actions are established as patterns over time, and they become recognisable as behaviours and reactions which are associated with circumstances and personalities.

The embryo is termed a foetus by the ninth week of gestation, and development adheres to a unique genetic pathway. Intervention in the pre-birth context is common if a previous sibling has been supported by social work or the parent has been referred to family services by health. The Family Nurse Partnership refer many teenage parents to our service, and it is often the case that the mothers and fathers are care-leavers (The Family Nurse Partnership, 2011).

Anxiety and depression are regarded as the most common mental-health problems pre-birth and post-birth, and mental-health status is often confirmed on a referral form with a diagnosis by a general practitioner. I observe

DOI: 10.4324/9781003358107-4

that young teenage parents describe these conditions frequently during child-protection conferences and present mental health as an explanation for inadequate parenting skills, aggression towards service-providers, and limited engagement with an action plan. Older parents tend to describe short-term negative feelings which are related to childhood abuse. I feel that society has become conversant with mental-health issues, particularly during this COVID-19 pandemic, and, in my experience, the younger generation of parents appear to seek medical support more readily than older peers. These reflections are simply based upon anecdotal evidence from my workplace, and I appreciate that interpretation of mental-health issues may vary in different racial and environmental cultures, even throughout the city of Glasgow. I work in a multicultural setting, and parents' attitudes and beliefs on these issues are formed through many different influences.

Exposure of an adversity by the media is useful, and in recent years domestic violence and support mechanisms have been publicised to and by governments, funding bodies, and victims. Domestic violence is a recurrent aspect of referrals to our service and often includes violence from teenage boys to their mothers. As a long-serving practitioner in a community service, I can usually recall the teenage boys as infants in the nursery playrooms. These circumstances present me with a realistic illustration and rationale for ante-natal care, pre-birth assessment in child protection, and early intervention for mother, father, and baby.

Foetal alcohol syndrome disorders are the greatest single cause of learning disability, and during COVID-19 lockdown periods the consumption of alcohol by local service-users increased, in comparison to drug use. Poverty and availability of substance supply contributes to the source of negative influences upon the unborn child. I clearly recall working in the 1980s in Glasgow as glue-sniffing and inhalation of shoe polish had a major destructive impact upon the mental health and physical well-being of young people. This substance misuse occurred in a context of high unemployment, perceived inequalities, and youth disaffection. Bronfenbrenner's bio-ecological systems of human development (Bronfenbrenner, 1979) gives great depth and clarity to understanding positive and negative direct, and indirect influences, from the strategic level of governments to the micro-systems of families and individual relationships.

I have worked with many babies who spend the first 18 months of life coping with withdrawal symptoms from parental drug use. Their little bodies arch with distress, and high-pitched crying depicts emotional and physical pain as the babies desperately attempt to seek solace from the effects. It is challenging for parents, and foster-carers, to understand and to respond to the cues of babies who are withdrawing from drug or alcohol abuse. The new little human body is confused and fighting to live within the context of traumatic influences. The baby is solely focused upon the physical effects, and emotional comfort is often rejected as his energy and motivation are given to coping with internal negative impact upon his well-being, and survival.

Reflective functioning and responsive care are often difficult attributes to acquire and to demonstrate by parents who are affected with drug usage. The health and well-being of parents need to be established before a baby can be given adequate parental support. Mother and baby residential rehabilitation facilities can provide useful environmental contexts to encourage change, but returning to a home community, and maintaining progress, are challenging for families.

Fonagy (1999) discussed the long-term effect of trauma upon relationships in childhood and adulthood. A child who experiences adversity does not have the benefit of a positive relationship role model to use throughout his lifespan. The context encompasses negative effects upon his reflective capacity and development of a sense of self. Illustration is based upon the child inhibiting his capacity to mentalise traumatic circumstances. The lack of understanding can lead to the child actively seeking support from an abuser, which Fonagy (1999) indicates as a need for physical contact.

The attachment system is activated within a context of trauma and abuse, and a consequence is chaotic attachment. Behaviours relating to an inherent desire for secure attachment prompt negative and inconsistent abusive actions of a perpetrator. A child's instinct is protection of himself emotionally and physically in the context of adversity. Findings from the study by Fonagy (1999) give four reasons for abuse impacting negatively upon the reflective functioning of a child in the earliest years and throughout his adulthood. This research was based upon data collection from adult participants who had low levels of reflective capacity.

1   If a child acknowledges the negative intentions of an abusive parent, then he views himself as worthless. The research indicates that a child who has low mentalisation capacity will interpret the behaviour of others by focusing upon the consequences: abuse which is directed to himself.

2   The child may gain a distorted view of reality which is based upon the abusive parent's interpretations.

3   The child may have minimal exposure to positive external influences from the world outside his immediate family.

4   The family atmosphere may negatively impact upon his reflective capacity which affects interpretation and comprehension of his sense of self. The child may link his emotional arousal with negative interaction or even abandonment. Consequently, the child limits his emotional reactions or adopts the parent's internal state within his own sense of self. Raised levels of cortisol may also contribute to neurodevelopmental abnormalities and a reduction in mentalisation.

Fonagy (1999) linked personality disorder in adulthood to individuals who had rejected a caregiver's abusive tendencies in childhood. This coping mechanism can lead to a child directly inhibiting mentalisation; thus, abuse in the early years can delay or impair development of a sense of the autobiographical self. In a context of normal development, integration of skills supports the child to mentalise his behaviour. However, in a context of personality disorder, the ability to use reflective functioning is diminished due to *fractionation* of these skills. Maltreatment activates the attachment system, but the context of abuse by a potential attachment figure results in disorganised or chaotic attachment.

Fonagy (1999) emphasised the domination of non-reflective internal working models within the relationships of individuals who have personality disorders. Uneven adaptation occurs as the mentalising resources are split between the external world and influences of others and the internal world of the individual's own mental state and comprehension of his sense of self. The research states that chaotic attachment emerges from a disorganised sense of self in which the child feels vulnerable and unsafe due to the negative internal representation of himself. He has limited reflective capacity.

Parents may respond to an infant's distress by a demonstration of fear or presentation of behaviour that induces fear within an infant. Explanation of these circumstances relates to the parent's inability to view the infant as an intentional mental being. The result is the infant's association with fear and lack of care in response to his emotional arousal. Over time, the child may adopt and demonstrate a similar dissociative response to his parent, and others. The participants in this research by Fonagy (1999) were adults who had personality disorders, and the researcher indicated palliative care as supporting development of the intentional mental self. The projected outcome is lessening of the gap between internal and external reality.

The rationale for this approach is also applied to intervention in the early years as a response to infant mental health. Emotional literacy has become a significant aspect of many curricula (Scottish Government, 2004), and nurture groups, or therapeutic play that promotes development of the intentional self in young children (Bratton et al. 2006).

Targeted interventions

Targeted interventions are available to families who are deemed to be "at risk" during pregnancy and post-birth. An identified outcome is to support reconfiguration of the child's internal working model. Parent–child support programmes can be effective in enabling the parent to view her child as an intentional mental agent and promoting the sense of self to the child. Immaturity in these areas can be exhibited as an unstable sense of self and impulsivity, which Fonagy (1999) associated with lack of emotional awareness, and the predominance of physical reactions in response to stress.

These programmes are often implemented through home visiting by health workers. Indicated interventions can be accessed for women who experience issues that are detrimental to the mother and unborn baby. Many interventions are twofold and support mentalisation and resolving past trauma, in addition to development of positive parenting, secure attachment, and healthy lifestyles. A bridge is created between internal and external reality for the child, and opportunities for imaginative play, supported by a secure attachment figure, can enrich this stage of development.

Researchers from Harvard University recently published an action guide for policy-makers, in 2020, which indicates three key messages regarding influences upon child development: adult–child relationships, early experiences, and environmental exposure (National Scientific Council on the Developing Child, 2020). Prior research (Siegel, 2003) highlighted the interaction between these influences and social-emotional development throughout the lifespan, specifically from the prenatal period to three years of age. These influences have a profound impact upon long-term health and well-being as foundations for healthy functioning systems are established.

A pregnant mother's stress, lack of nutrition, and environmental exposure can result in the child having an increased risk of heart disease, obesity, diabetes, and mental-health conditions. Anxiety, hypervigilance, and depression affect development and impact upon the emergence of systemic properties, for example, mobility and communication skills. Chronic negative influences can contribute to a cycle in which the child's resilience is reduced and he becomes more susceptible to future adverse influence. Pathological outcomes may result if a child's understanding of himself is detrimentally affected (Siegel, 2003).

Siegel (2003) described the mind as a complex system that encompassed many layers and potential connections which were influenced by genetics, environment, and time. Mental health is regarded as a self-organising process that supports an individual to achieve maximum complexity. If the system does not progress towards complexity, then it is regarded as experiencing stress. The complexity of this system emerges from two fundamental processes, termed "differentiation" and "integration". Differentiation relates to specialisation of components and integration to the forming of a whole system. A functional link is created by neural integration which occurs as differentiated circuits in the brain form a coherent information-processing system.

Complexity

Therapeutic relationships, whether in a formal context of psychotherapy or informal interactions, can enable self-organisation of the mind to progress towards complexity. Siegel (2003) stated that human minds are created through neural functioning, and this researcher identified 12 aspects that feature in therapeutic relationships and support organisation of the mind: connection, compassion, contingency, cohesion, continuity, coherence, clarity, co-construction, complexity, consciousness, creativity, and community. The mind is a subjective entity that evolves over the lifespan in accordance with influences from genetics, environment, relationships, and personality. There are patterns of flow in the mind that involve energy and information. These patterns can occur intra-personally and inter-personally. Ultimately, the mind can alter the brain and the brain alter the mind as a result of information-processing (Siegel, 2003).

Neural integration refers to the different elements of the brain, or processing modalities, functioning as a whole entity (Siegel, 2003). As neurons are activated then patterns of brain activity emerge which are consolidated and extended during common *or* repeated experiences. Practitioners will observe similar actions and emotions in infants during daily drop-off and pick-up times that become established as routines. Personality and well-being affect infants to a greater degree than children and adults. As humans mature then their ability and capacity to overcome personal inclination and to adhere to social expectations increases.

The young child relies on a consistent secure attachment relationship to direct his learning. Over a period of time, the child is able to function independently by referring to memories created by this essential relationship. Informal interactions occur between parent and child on multiple occasions throughout every day and night. Practitioners can support parents by highlighting the importance of constructing communication pathways with a young child to nurture development and to form secure attachment. Therapeutic progress is often expressed as an increase in creativity. In nurseries, children may not participate in arts and crafts activities or imaginative play for several weeks after the induction period. A child needs time to feel liberated from his perceived emotional and social barriers in order to express his inner thoughts and ideas through creative play.

The parent's own experiences of attachment relationships in early childhood impact upon the care of subsequent generations. In 2003, a team of researchers concluded a 23-year longitudinal study, and the findings focused upon a concept termed "earned secure attachment" (Roisman et al., 2003). This research explored the potential changes in understanding and demonstration of attachment in adults who had described childhood relationships with their parents as insecure. The descriptor "earned secure" referred to the increase in the adults' ability and capacity to experience and to express secure attachment with their own children. This ability was realised for many of the participants, and secure attachment was established with the second generation.

Brain development includes a process of pruning. This emotive and descriptive term refers to negative impact upon synaptic growth in which neural connections may be not form due to minimal or no activation, and some neurons die. The pruning process is particularly activated during adolescent years. Activation is dependent on genetic timing of growth in these circuits in addition to experience or activity-dependent development.

The infant/child's interaction with the environment, and relationships, is influenced by genetic coding and determines developmental pathways. Memory is a major catalyst to development. For example, a visual/pictorial or text prompt to the retina activates the optic nerve, and the information traverses to the left side of the brain towards the communication-processing area. Memory is one of the neural processes that benefits from repetition to increase the likelihood of neurons linking together on more than one occasion. Memory can cause prior experiences and accompanying emotions which are associated with a specific prompt to be recalled and to assimilate with a new experience. Siegel (2003) described integration of experiences within one person's brain being influenced by the flow from another person's brain. Knowledge and understanding of influences upon integration provides a rationale for implementation of learning being supported by an adult or peer.

Care plans, and regular observation and assessment of each child by a key worker, facilitate effective curriculum delivery within a service. In addition, recall is used to support children's skill in reflecting upon past events, gaining awareness of memory storage by focusing upon internal thoughts, experiencing these processes, and expressing personal interpretation. The recall and discussion of positive experiences creates a useful initial stepping stone to children accessing memories and understanding their actions and emotions. One example relates to a child's memory of nursery activities from the previous day.

Reference to previous experiences provides an opportunity for a carer to recall the child's actions in detail and to create a vivid picture by using relevant and realistic prompts to support the child's reflective capacity. Reflection upon prior experiences which have not been observed by a key worker, for example a birthday party in the home environment, provide opportunities for the practitioner to use questions as prompts and to explore the memory alongside a child. These scenarios appoint control of the situation to a child and increase his mastery. Conversing with an infant or young child is an art form and requires skills in empathising with others, accurate observation and assessment of needs and emotions, and responses based upon reflection and interpretation.

Neural development

The mind and brain are regulated by the following:

1   Internal constraints and facilitators in the form of synaptic connections between neurons. These barriers and enhancers to development can change quickly over time.
2   External constraints and facilitators, which include experiences from the proximal and distal environments, relationships, and communication skills.

The infant or young child's mental health has a direct impact on his capacity to self-regulate emotions and actions. Siegel (2003) used the term "two-person governed self-regulation" to described support strategies from an adult or peer to a child. Initially, these strategies can alter external influences and thereafter contribute to reconfiguration of the child's inner working model. Relationships can change the physiological aspect of neural connections within the brain of each person. Neuroplasticity is significant to development (Doidge, 2008). Connections support self-regulation and contribute to achievement of complexity and, ultimately, good mental health. This optimum outcome from a secure attachment relationship in early childhood can continue to be achieved whether the attachment figure is present in person or within the child's implicit memories.

During the first three years of life, development of the right hemisphere of the brain dominates neural growth. This right side is responsible for processing non-verbal communications, for example, tone or gestures, facial expressions, emotion, and social cognition, which relates to theory of mind. The theory of mind entails a child understanding that other people have opinions, thoughts, and emotions that differ from his own. I have often heard lay terms used colloquially that demonstrate comprehension of this concept from the perspective of parents or grandparents, "He is putting his thoughts together. He is using joined-up thinking. He can sense what other people are thinking. Both sides of the brain are talking to each other." These are phrases I regularly hear from families during parenting work, and it is easy to capitalise upon these thoughts to promote the significance of a parent's input to a child's neural development.

The left side of the brain develops at a later stage than the right side, and it uses syllogistic reasoning. This type of reasoning encompasses cause and effect, and it contributes toward the development of self as a teleological agent (Whitters, 2019). The left side of the brain relies on information from the right side to create coherent narratives in order to understand sequences of events and, ultimately, lead to neural integration between the left and right hemispheres of the brain. The brain follows an innate tendency to seek out complexity of processes by integration, differentiation, and regulation.

Barriers to these processes may include short-term stress responses or long-term post-traumatic stress disorder. Additionally, research indicates potential for damage to the corpus callosum which connects the two hemispheres (Teicher et al., 2002). The corpus callosum consists of bands of neural tissue that support information transfer. Damaged connections have also been related to shrinking of the hippocampus which can affect a child's ability to develop and to use explicit memory.

Findings from research have linked damage of this neural area to child abuse and neglect (Teicher et al., 2002) and association with excessive toxic hormone secretion as a result of stressful experiences. Too much cortisol can cause death of neuron cells. The hippocampus has cortisol receptors that increase vulnerability to the impact of stress. This area of the brain does not fully form until 16–18 months of age, which is a period when the child starts to use explicit memory (Siegel, 2003). These milestones of development signify the importance of early intervention by practitioners, parents, society, and governments.

Therapeutic support delivered within a secure relationship can instigate connections between the two hemispheres. Emotion influences all neural circuits and, subsequently, mental functioning. The amygdala processes emotions, which results in the child's internal experience of an emotion, his expression of this sensation to the outside world, and his perception of emotions in others. It is known that the face-recognition cells within the amygdala are activated by facial representation of emotions in others. Daily encounters between a parent/carer and infant provide multiple opportunities to support links between the two hemispheres.

It is important for parents and practitioners to appreciate the power of any interaction to reduce the impact of stress upon learning and development. Many services will implement formal therapeutic interventions to families, but daily play and home/nursery routines also present rich and stimulating environments. Multi-modal approaches can target different learning styles of families and can respond sensitively to increasing capacity and ability as time progresses. Broad experiences throughout play activate the child's genes which results in protein production and changes to the architecture of the brain as new synapses form. Experiences gained from play also change brain function.

Promoting attachment

We continue to wear COVID-19 protection face masks at drop-off and pick-up time, and, contrary to expectations, secure attachment is established between infants and carers. It is never too late to promote attachment relationships with children. Research by Siegel (2003) outlined five approaches that contribute to secure attachment if actioned by parents: contingent communication, reflective dialogue, repair following rupture of the relationship, emotional communication, and coherent narratives.

These approaches can change the neural connections as described by the following examples.

1 **Contingent communication**: The parent notices the infant signalling, interprets the message, and responds in a timely and sensitive manner. The infant is waiting for a response, and he embraces the message because it is attuned to his needs and interests at a point of time. The infant uses the parent's response to develop his own perception of the situation then sends another signal to his parent; thus, the cycle continues. I often observe parents and children during daily encounters as they interact with stimuli which includes the parent's face or pram artefacts. Contingent communication prevails. Contingent communication has a predominant cultural element, and it immerses the infant in a lifestyle relating to his family. Family-based culture includes beliefs, needs, interests, and the characteristics that give every family a unique identity.

2 **Reflective dialogue**: Contingent communication as used for babies in their earliest years develops with the addition of verbal dialogue. The parent is no longer reflecting the infant's needs in isolation but extending knowledge and understanding in relation to self and others. The parent introduces the infant to a communication medium through this dialogue.

3 **Repair**: Ruptures in relationships can occur often in relation to issues of tiredness, prioritising attention, and tasks, limit setting, poor health, and

stress of a parent. Repair entails acknowledgement of the infant's needs, information on mitigating circumstances that have caused the rupture, and a route to repair. It is always useful for children to learn that a parent, and others, may not always be able to attune affectively, but a strong consistent attachment relationship can create a repair bridge.

4 **Emotional communication**: Supporting a child to experience and to cope with negative emotions is equally as important as rejoicing and celebrating the positives. The child begins to gain self-control, regulation, and resilience for the occasions when he is dealing with adversities without direct support from an attachment figure.

5 **Coherent narratives**: Storytelling between parent and child can greatly support the creation of coherent narratives of family events, and circumstances, in addition to issues external to the household. These narratives broaden the child's knowledge, prompt imagination, contribute to explicit memory coding opportunities, and create multiple interpersonal bonding experiences for parent and child. My work with families who are affected by internal trauma, and adverse lifestyles, responds to immaturity in areas of social and emotional development, particularly from birth to three years of age. Monthly observations of each infant, and records which many parents keep of significant milestones, demonstrate areas in which development is steady, plateaued, or delayed. It is important to target areas of strength in order to provide a framework for holistic development.

The orbitofrontal cortex is behind the orbit of the eyes. This is a key location in the brain that facilitates the cortex's role in neural integration. Coordination occurs between the cortex, limbic structures, and the brain stem, and impacts upon mental health and repairing the effects of trauma. Schore (1994) identified a function of the orbitofrontal cortex as regulation of the autonomic nervous system that controls heart rate, respiration, and intestines. The two branches are termed:

1 The sympathetic branch, which speeds up processes.
2 The parasympathetic branch, which slows down processes.

Short- or long-term effects upon the effective functioning of the orbitofrontal region can lead to a sensation of disconnection from the proximal environment and difficulty in reflecting upon self. Practical consequences can result in an infant or child being unable to give direct eye contact to another person, despite an available nurturing attachment figure. This results from emotional influences upon the infant rather than a physical restriction. The behaviour may be interpreted incorrectly as an infant or child choosing to be inattentive and to reject relationships. It may well be that the child is creating a barrier to a relationship due to the effects of prior trauma and implicit memories of similar overtures from adults in his adverse lifestyle.

Stress

Coates (2010) investigated the neuroendocrine system in a context of adverse childhood experiences and the impact of stress in adulthood. This system comprises interaction between the brain, nervous system, and hormones, and it regulates emotions and stress responses. Findings indicated a long-term impact of adversity linked to disruption in the neuroendocrine system which altered the hypothalamic-pituitary-adrenocortical. The state of hyper-arousal may persist during the lifespan as the body remains primed for a flight or fight reaction. Fear is experienced and regarded as relative to current influences, although it originates from past events. Additionally, trauma response tendencies can be acquired from one generation to another through copying and learned behaviours.

The study by Coates (2010) clearly describes the brain's reaction to stress.

- The limbic system is composed of a network of neural cells that encompasses the amygdala and hippocampus.
- This area of the brain controls emotions in relation to survival and activates a response to threat.
- Threat causes the amygdala to release hormones in preparation for fight, flight, or freeze responses.
- Emotions are processed by the amygdala prior to information being registered by the cortex.
- The hippocampus supports information to be processed and passed to the cortex.
- The hippocampus can be affected adversely by hormones, and functioning ability may decrease.
- The volume of the hippocampus can be reduced in a context of environmental stress and associated with negative emotional states of dissociation, panic, anxiety, and poor memory.
- The cortex is the outer layer of the brain which relates to cognition, and messages are passed from limbic system to cortex.
- Problem-solving occurs in the front area of the cortex and learning which relates to experience takes place in the prefrontal cortex.

Potential threat is registered within the fast tracts of the limbic system. The information which is passed to the prefrontal cortex may not be sufficient for an infant to differentiate between an actual or a perceived threat, and he may misinterpret stimuli and appear to overreact (Coates, 2010). Carers are familiar with children overreacting to minor issues, and this explanation by Coates provides comprehension of these processes which supports intervention and responsive practice within daily routines.

The left side of the brain is responsible for perception and expression of language, and interpretation of circumstances. The right side of the brain has responsibility for perception and expression of emotions. Research has indicated a negative impact upon development of the left side of the brain in a context of adverse childhood experiences. A research study found that verbal abuse from parents can be associated with lack of development in areas of the left hemisphere of the brain that process language (Choi et al., 2008) in addition to negative impact upon the tracts linked with emotional regulation. This study accessed data from 1,271 healthy young adults who were initially screened for exposure to childhood adversity. Fractional anisotropy was investigated, and three white matter tract regions on the left side of the brain indicated a significant reduction compared to the norm. Findings associated the differences in fractional anisotropy with the level of maternal verbal abuse and potential effect upon language development in addition to evidence of psychopathology. These findings are informative by publicising the negative impact of ridicule, humiliation, and disdain upon brain connectivity.

Teicher et al. (2004) conducted a neural study in which child abuse was shown to affect development of the corpus callosum by limiting growth. The right and left hemisphere of the brain are connected through this corpus callosum and interact with one another in a context of neural processing. Findings indicated that neglect had a high association with this reduction in growth, and sexual abuse was specifically linked with smaller corpus callosum in girls. Participant group was composed of 25 girls and 26 boys. A smaller corpus callosum resulted in reduced integration between left and right hemisphere and noticeable changes in mood or personality. Intervention was recommended by Rothschild (2000) as a means to lower stress hormones and to maintain healthy functioning of the hippocampus.

Memory was investigated in a study by McClelland (1998). Findings indicated that explicit memory, based upon stimuli from the environment, had a series of stages that supported the retention of information. The first stage of the brain registering an experience lasts for under half a second, and it involves input to sensory memory. During the second stage, which lasts for about 30 seconds, the information is deposited within working memory. The third stage may incur days, months, or years, as the information is retained in long-term memory. The final stage is the consolidation of long-term memories into permanent memory which may take days or months to be completed. Permanent memory is independent of the hippocampus.

It is informative that the study by McClelland (1998) raised sleep as an important contributing factor to these memory processes. Health visitors, midwives, social workers, and early years practitioners have an essential role to play in educating parents about the reason for establishing healthy sleep patterns appropriate to an infant's age, physiological needs, and personality. I find that parents are keen to understand sleep patterns in their children, and it is intriguing to learn about our brains working hard during sleep periods to process and to retain information.

Research has identified evidence of stress responses in the foetus before birth (Gunnar & Barr, 1998). Cortisol is known to impact physiologically and psychologically upon the development of the foetus and subsequently upon behaviour during childhood. Outcomes associated with antenatal anxiety include premature delivery, low birthweight (Association of Infant Mental Health United Kingdom, 2021), and difficulty in creating an attachment bond. These challenges may stem from a mother's negative representation of her baby before the birth which is created within a context of stress and high anxiety.

The COVID-19 pandemic is a current stress upon infant mental health through the mother's experience of direct and indirect adversities. A survey conducted in 2020 identified two main causes of stress which occurred during the first wave of the pandemic: participants felt unprepared for the birth and fearful of infection from COVID-19. Poverty was also cited as an influential factor to a high level of stress which was experienced by mothers during this time (Association of Infant Mental Health United Kingdom, 2021). Digital media were described by parents as useful means of communication which could be accessed at opportune times. Participants identified positive outcomes from the digital media as choices in response to needs at a point of time and privacy to share information in this learning context.

Environmental stress factors lead to a fight, flight, or freeze reaction that can impact upon the following bodily systems.

- The brain and nervous system, which manage and respond to stress factors.
- The heart and cardiovascular system, which distribute oxygen throughout the body within the blood.
- The gut and metabolic system, which transform food into energy for the body.
- The immune system, which defends against disease, and also supports healing of injuries.
- The neuroendocrine system, which maintains the balance of hormones.

The Harvard study (National Scientific Council on the Developing Child, 2020) concluded that policy-makers should implement programmes of intervention that reduce daily stresses and toxic exposure within the environment and provide support in the earliest prenatal stages. Daily stresses are cited as poverty, community racism, a lack of suitable housing, and ongoing food insecurity. Community programmes can react to issues within a local area, and implementation strategies can be responsive to needs and culture of the residents, for example, food banks and second-hand clothing stores.

Learning and development

Vygotsky (1978) studied the processes of learning and development in a context of socio-cultural theory. This theorist termed learning as a higher process which is integrated with development from birth. Inherent human psychological functions mature and develop in accordance with genetic timetabling relating to growth. Consistent growth requires a regular source of food, rest, and stimulating learning opportunities.

These functions are influenced by family and community culture and expectations of society and may support or hinder realisation of developmental potential. Vygotsky (1978) concluded that learning was not regarded as development per se, but it was a process that accompanied development and enabled it to occur. He proposed two developmental levels with the descriptors of "actual" and "potential", which indicated that one level was achieved and the second level *could be achieved* if nurtured by influences responsive to the circumstances.

- Actual developmental level: achieved through independent problem-solving. Quantitative scales may be used to determine a child's actual developmental level in comparison to the norm of a particular chronological age.
- Potential developmental level: achieved through an increase in problem-solving skill which is guided by adults or more capable peers. The potential level of attainment is higher than the actual developmental level. Qualitative methods are generally used to record this level of attainment. Professional observations and direct involvement with a child's interactions provide insight into evidence of a higher level of skill through application.

The zone of proximal development, as termed by Vygotsky (1978), is regarded as the distance between actual development (retrospective) and potential development (prospective). Actual development relates to an outcome which is already achieved, and potential development encompasses a successive stage of learning in which an outcome is not necessarily predetermined. It is not always easy for an adult to establish if a child has achieved his initial goal or been diverted to a different goal through internal or external factors. This process incurs divergent thinking.

The popular educational approach of child-led play provides opportunities for children to use creativity and imaginative thinking, although play occurs within an environment implemented by adults. Consideration of a zone of proximal development by an educator can enhance the learning experience by removing the constriction and potential limitation of predetermined goals, particularly within a service in which the pedagogy is bound by curricular outcomes. Comprehension of child development and learning processes liberates the educator to reflect upon each child's potential and to maintain delivery of a curriculum in a context of responsive and inclusive teaching.

Language functions as an interpersonal and intrapersonal aid to the acquisition of knowledge and understanding. Language facilitates communication between peers and adults, and it can be used to incite a child's curiosity by indicating further learning through scaffolding of ideas. Language also provides a tool for internal thoughts and ideas to be processed and compared to prior knowledge. Finally, language supports consolidation or reconfiguration of the inner working model.

Copying is a common source of learning which is often described within a context of the mirror neuron system, particularly in the earliest years. The theory of mind is dependent on this skill and usually develops by the age of four or five years. This significant stage also contributes to socialising effectively within a society, and Cicchetti and Toth (2006) described the process as a shift from situation-based to representation-based understanding of behaviour. The following outcomes emerge from the theory of mind.

- Ability (intellectual) and capacity (emotional well-being) to self-regulate actions.
- Knowledge and understanding of the link between actions and behaviour.
- The ability to differentiate and to understand emotions and context and to communicate emotions through language or other media – emotional literacy.
- The capacity to demonstrate empathic responding to the needs of others.

Humans are products of culture and contributors to propagation of family, community, and national culture throughout each generation. Language or alternative communication skills are integral to development, and verbal intercourse provides a medium for transferring family, community, or societal culture to a learner. The concept of culture includes knowledge, understanding, attitudes, values, and beliefs. These aspects can guide the child's actions and reactions to the world in a manner that reflects his local context and contributes to formation of his sense of self in the earliest years.

Tronick and Beeghly (2011) linked infant mental health to a young child's level of understanding. In childhood, comprehension is gained through play. Vygotsky (1978) explored the concept of play from a theoretical perspective. He proposed that babies and infants seek and expect the fulfilling of needs within a short time frame; therefore, the time gap between desire and fulfilment is brief. Vygotsky assimilates play and imagination by presenting the two issues together as he describes the actions and experiences of children over three years of age. Imagination is termed a new psychological process at this early stage of development.

Therapeutic and generic play provide a safe context for children to identify their interests, to express their personalities, to change their ideas quickly or over time, and to use imagination to fulfil unrealistic objectives. Play also supports children to emulate daily observations of life in practice and to experiment and develop skills safely within an arena that has limited repercussions. Repercussions relate to the imposition of social rules, and consequences that contribute to the creation of a safe play space and necessary boundaries to exploration for a young learner. During a child's early years of development, the breaking of friendships or negative communications with carers can affect his self-confidence, albeit on a temporary and fluctuating basis.

A young child's behaviour can indicate over-responsiveness in which he seeks high-intensity movement. Examples are climbing, hanging upside down, and risk-taking that may be misinterpreted as aggressive defiance to social and physical boundaries. The child may appear agitated as he attempts to conform to expectations of behaviour, for example, biting his sleeve, moving his legs during periods of sitting, and drumming his fingers. Alternatively, a young child may demonstrate under-responsiveness and appear defensive to touch, express apathy, and fail to notice changes or stimulation in the environment. The child may have a poor sense of direction and immature sequencing memory.

The early years environment

Every childcare and education student will learn why and how to set up a variety of learning environments. However, over time I have observed that practitioners develop favourite personalised approaches to setting up a playroom. The rationale is not clear, the curricular links are not easy to detect or to action, and aesthetic presentation can take prominence for the practitioner. The following section highlights playroom areas or stations, the rationale, outcomes, and key points for implementation. It is noted that the provision of an adult space within each area is a significant contributory factor to creation and maintenance of a secure attachment relationship between key worker and child.

- Physical: indoors and outdoors.
- Arts and crafts: creative, water, sand.
- Imaginative: small world, home corner.
- Table-top.
- Literacy and book corner.
- Floor play.

Physical

Rationale: To understand physical and emotional self.
Outcome: Gross motor skills, balance, proprioception, spatial awareness, social rules, sequencing, action, and reaction.

- Proprioception may be termed body awareness and relates to the child's knowledge and understanding of the interaction between his skeleton and muscles and control of his physical movements.
- Spatial awareness is the child's knowledge and understanding of environmental structures, spaces, and how to negotiate his body around the play area.

Key points of implementation: Health and safety for individual and group, risk assessment in response to children's maturity, attraction, stimulation, consolidation and extension, adult space.

Arts and crafts

Rationale: To understand physical, emotional, and social self.
Outcome: Fine motor skills, hand-to-eye coordination, sensory awareness, science concepts, numerical concepts, action, and reaction.
Key points of implementation: Variety of choices, variety of media, personal and group space, adult space.

Imaginative

Rationale: Play that represents own world or imaginary world, social and emotional self.
Outcome: Conceptual understanding of the world, understanding of personal impact upon the world.
Key points of implementation: Accessible individually or group, comfortable, appropriate choices, adult space.

Table-top

Rationale: Cognitive skills, sequencing, solitary/parallel/cooperative play
Outcome: Memory, hand-to-eye coordination, scaffolding learning, seeking support – peers or adult.
Key points of implementation: Attractive, accessible, stimulating, adult space.

Literacy and book corner

Rationale: Literacy and emotional literacy, opportunity for down-regulation.
Outcome: Fine motor skills, sequencing, link word and text, imaginative skills, memory, rest.
Key points of implementation: Attractive, accessible, stimulating, adult space

Floor play

Rationale: Sense of physical, social, emotional, and teleological self, cognitive skills.
Outcome: Fine and gross motor skills, action, and reaction, increase resilience, problem-solving.
Key points of implementation: Attractive, accessible, safe, combining several choices of media, adult space.

Lack of opportunity for physical development can induce passivity, and it can result in the brain existing in a neurologically neutral state. The passive child may appear to have a high level of well-being, but his cognitive and emotional development are limited by the proximal environment. A readiness to learn leads to behaviour in which the infant actively seeks out knowledge and identifies opportunities to explore, despite limited stimulation. Good mental and physical health are important and include the meeting of basic needs, for example, food, water, and personal hygiene. The availability of an attachment figure and opportunities that provide predictability, consistency, and repeatability contribute to a child's readiness to learn. Explicit memories are formed from the environmental experience, and implicit memories are created by the emotions that accompany the child's explorations and interactions with others.

Self-control is usually high during free play as the young child is using developing skills associated with his imagination, and he begins to develop abstract thought. Objects can be transformed for different purposes, initially within the child's imagination then followed by actions that specifically relate to the child's interests, needs, and knowledge of the world. Vygotsky (1978) expressed that a preschool child's actions are led by his ideas as opposed to his reaction and interactions with concrete objects. A child may previously have demonstrated subordination to social rules; however, during free-play episodes, a child can experience pleasure and fulfilment. The child can change rules and take control of his own actions. The child's perceptions of his proximal and distal world change. The child achieves mastery and power, which can increase his resilience to life's adversities; however, distraction within the external environment can rapidly reduce a child's involvement and well-being.

Box 4.1 Example from practice

The early morning mist had cleared, and a pale autumn sunshine was peeping over the horizon. The horizon in this scene was the distant backdrop of Glasgow city centre, which made an impact statement through a vision of slim church spires stretching high into the watery blue sky. I transferred my gaze from the vista to my immediate environment of a city community nursery. I was perched on the edge of a log fence which was designed to be eco-friendly and to promote an aesthetic space within the concrete play setting, but it was not so comfortable for conducting my professional task.

I considered my role for today. I had come to this early years service to observe 4-year-old Zeeshan as a prelude to implementing therapeutic intervention. The little preschool boy had been referred by his family and nursery staff as emotionally immature and displaying challenging behaviour. A perceptive line within the referral form by the boy's key worker had tentatively suggested that a higher ability than peers was emerging; however, the final referral comment had conclusively stated, "Zeeshan will not cope well in school at this stage of his development."

The council referral form boxed the child's behaviour into tight compartments, and the word "concerns" was highlighted in bold black print and featured within each section heading of the referral. An easy copy and paste for the creator of this communication and a concept that leads the writer and reader to focus upon negative interpretation of Zeeshan's involvement with his learning arenas.

Considering the presentation of information upon a referral form is insightful to the professional as each word is heavily laden with nuance, implications, and emotion that tell a child's story from a carer's perspective. A record of information can be useful in communicating a professional's or carer's interpretation and understanding of a child's needs. The conclusive statement indicated to me that referrers had placed the responsibility of integrating within the school environment upon the 4-year-old boy.

As I study the written record of Zeeshan, I am gradually creating visual images of the way in which his interactions are portrayed, and responded to, by his parents and early years educators. A picture emerges of Zeeshan's behaviour, and it is clear that mention is not made of his needs. Behaviour is a child's communication with the world that has a rationale based upon need. Behaviour reveals emotions, strengths, weaknesses, and fears. Behaviour can represent a child's plea for help to interpret and to respond to the trials of childhood. Challenging behaviour emerges from a gap in a child's development which may relate to a limitation of input from an adult, or ability and capacity to learn. Identification of the referrer is significant too, and it relays the source of concern from a parent or professional perspective.

The rationale of my observation was Zeeshan's perspective of the world in addition to his preferred mode of learning and communication strategies. The play space was adorned with the ubiquitous outdoor equipment used by early years teams throughout the world: bikes, tyres, wooden ramps, weather shelters, and balls. An indication of a nurture corner was displayed by a large green and yellow tartan rug which was scattered with a few books and large purple beanbags. I could see that Zeeshan was restless and dissatisfied with the play choices. As I watched quietly from my wooden perch, the tall 4-year-old started to jump up and down on the spot. His arms were held flat against his sides and head held high.

Zeeshan increased the height of his pogo jumps, and I noticed that he shook each hand sharply downwards, and he maintained the beat of this play by flicking his wrists. He appeared to relish the sense of achievement. Suddenly Zeeshan stopped. A few plastic drainpipes had been laid invitingly at angles to one another and set alongside a box of little hard balls. Zeeshan approached with caution then quickly he made his plan of action. Pipes were constructed at various descending heights, and a little crowd of peers gathered to watch respectfully. A young girl explored alongside Zeeshan, near to his play space but not integrated into a peer dyad. Rebecca favoured the smallest yellow balls and quickly gathered them together as Zeeshan drew nearer to her domain.

Zeeshan placed an orange ball into the top pipe with purposeful intent, and the group held their breath and watched. Zeeshan cocked his head to one side as he listened to the ball tumbling from one pipe to another. The youngsters clapped and laughed; however, this response seemed to distract the 4-year-old constructor, and Zeeshan abruptly left the scene. A snapshot observation which was packed with information on Zeeshan's skills and needs. I scribbled furiously to record my notes as I considered the child's motivation, task focus, and creativity.

The clapping of peers had caused Zeeshan to leave the scene of the activity. This external influence affected the young boy's focus upon achieving his goal. Adaptability is a key skill in demonstration of creativity and imaginative play, especially within a social context of a busy nursery in which the pedagogy is child-led and often unpredictable.

Making meaning

The term "distance", as used by Vygotsky (1978), relates to the transitional phase of the child's intellectual capacity. A transition occurs as the child is supported by an adult or peer, and his knowledge and understanding increases to a higher degree than would have been achieved through independent play. Zeeshan and his peers transformed plastic pipes into a learning experience that portrayed understanding of height, weight, length, speed, and skill in eye–hand coordination. Once potential development is achieved then the new knowledge and understanding is assimilated by the child within his inner working model. Processes are internalised and thereafter encompassed within the capacity for independent achievement. This level of functioning is subsequently maintained without further adult or peer input. Vygotsky's law of double formation refers to these two levels of higher psychological functioning (Whitters, 2019).

The work by Tronick and Beeghly (2011) highlighted the enormity of bio-psychosocial processes which contribute to making meaning for an infant, and the core bio-psychosocial state of consciousness. Personality affects the infant's interactions with his world, and positive feedback can elicit emotions of joy and well-being. The cycle of learning commences at conception and continues throughout the entire lifespan.

Tronick and Beeghly (2011) also describe the making of meaning by infants as limiting engagement to specific areas, in addition to extending the infant's awareness of his role and ability within a family context. The infant's increase in understanding of his world impacts positively upon development, for example, physical skills and communication; however, influences may also affect development adversely. The study by these authors indicated that meanings that limit growth on a long-term basis increase the potential for pathological outcomes. An example of adverse childhood experience in infancy is a mother who is suffering from postnatal depression. The young baby may develop representation of himself as negative which results in withdrawal from active investigation and exploration of the environment or hypervigilance to perceived dangers. If the infant is exposed to a variety of stimulating opportunities for learning, then he will acquire resilience to negative impacts which promotes normative development.

Shonkoff et al. (2021) published research that focused upon the foundations of health, learning, and behaviour. Findings emphasised the significance of the perinatal period and infancy to brain development, the immune system, and metabolic regulation. The discussion includes the use of an interactive gene–environment–time framework to promote comprehension of the effects from adversities. Adversity deprives a child of physical, social, emotional, and intellectual stimulation and may additionally pose a direct threat to development (Asmussen et al. 2020).

The study by Shonkoff et al. (2021) indicates that health and development are influenced by interactive adaptations that commence prior to conception and continue throughout the lifespan. Impact factors that should be considered within a context of intervention by services include genetic predispositions. Genetic factors may be activated by physical and social environments, age, and, inextricably, the time period with regards to an infant or child's ability to uptake learning. An additional consideration is the sensitivity of the individual to a learning context, which often relates to personality, as described in the example from practice.

Another issue was raised by Schechter et al. (2019) as the stage of development in which the adversity was experienced. It is known that memory recall of events is apparent in infants during their first year of life, and by 24 months long-term memories can influence an infant's reactions and emotions. If an adversity is experienced prior to language development, then it can be difficult for a child to gain comprehension of these circumstances. There may be specific sensory triggers that remind the child of an adversity by influencing his body's reaction in a similar way to the initial source. A child may use dissociative processes to gain protection from his emotions, and this can affect memory recall and subsequent understanding of the issues.

One recent research study found that infants who demonstrated the greatest sensitivity to adversities were also the most responsive to intervention (Shonkoff et al., 2021). Impact factors can be used positively to reduce adversity, or the effects minimised in order to promote resilience. Stress is an example of an impact factor which is commonly categorised into three levels.

1   Positive stress is associated with a short-term physiological reaction which can be managed by the individual with the support of a responsive adult.
2   Tolerable stress also activates physiological reaction, for example, immune or metabolic responses. This category of stress is often associated with a particular event or trauma. The physiological impact can be reduced by an adult promoting the child's coping skills which increases his resilience.
3   Toxic stress can have a severe and long-lasting impact upon health and development. Frequent and prolonged activation of the stress response

system can result in permanent changes to neural connections, and biological systems. For example, increased inflammation and inability to regulate insulin levels. This category of stress is linked to circumstances in which a protective relationship is not available, or the adversities, and effects, are beyond control of the adults who are present. Poverty is often cited as a source of toxic stress. Furthermore, the available relationship itself may be the source of adversity. Shonkoff et al. (2021) advised that the source of stress is not the defining factor of toxicity, but it is the *duration* and *timing* of biological affects which can lead to an increase in chronic illness.

Responsive practice

Asmussen et al. (2020) suggested that an alteration in threat, reward, and memory-processing, as a result of adversity, could cause changes to children's social-emotional functioning. Consequently, these authors indicated that the changes may affect relationships with others, and cause carers and peers to reduce or to remove their supportive strategies.

Recommendations by Shonkoff et al. (2021) include supportive and responsive relationships for infants and children that reflect individual needs, reactions, and interactions within an environment. Additionally, family-centred learning promotes secure attachment between child and caregiver within a consistently nurturing context. Interventions can have a direct positive impact upon the cycle of negative parenting in response to endemic adversities and support a parent to improve self-regulation of herself and the child. Further recommendations advocated reduction of stress through economic and psychosocial interventions.

The study by Milot et al. (2016) of 33 neglected children and 72 non-neglected children, focused upon potential links between neglect, complex trauma, and short-term consequences. Key messages for practice include application of knowledge by the practitioner. This information is gained through in-depth assessment of trauma history within a case file and an understanding of the personal characteristics of child and parent. Trauma-informed practice encompasses provision of an environment in which each child feels safe, therapeutic intervention increases responsiveness of parents, and there is greater comprehension of links between emotions and behaviours of parent and child.

Interestingly, the previous authors (Shonkoff et al. 2021) also placed importance on a practitioner's use of normative values for infants and children in accordance with age and expected stage of development. Knowledge and understanding of developmental norms and projected outcomes support planning and implementation of intervention by services and may increase understanding of primary caregivers in the context of a home environment.

A public-health report was published in Scotland, in May 2020, just a few months after the first wave of COVID-19 pandemic, and the writer indicated that the long-term impact of coronavirus upon society is unknown at this stage (Hetherington, 2020). The pandemic is clearly recognised as an impactful adversity of the 21st century, and Hetherington described that a response should occur at community, family, and individual level, in addition to broader society. This author advocates a public-health approach that prevents or minimises children's adverse experiences during formative years. Public health focuses upon the needs of a population or specific groups, as opposed to a clinician's response to an individual. The study identifies social determinants of health as childhood experiences, housing, education, social support, family income, employment, community, and access to health services.

Hetherington (2020) describes three approaches to public health.

1   **Primary prevention**: Early intervention to prevent negative impact.
2   **Secondary prevention**: Early intervention to minimise negative impact.
3   **Tertiary prevention**: Intervention that directly responds to known negative impacts.

Ghosts in a nursery

The concept of ghosts in a nursery was presented in research which was conducted half a century ago (Fraiberg et al., 1975), and the understanding of these issues continues to have current relevance (Scottish Government & NHS Scotland, 2021). It is well known that parenting patterns are often learned and repeated between generations. Fraiberg and the research team described these ghosts as being expressed unconsciously within the parent–infant relationship.

The descriptor of unresolved parents (Fraiberg et al., 1975) is associated with the concept of ghosts in a nursery; however, current practice states that negative issues should not be used to define an individual's identity. Each organisation has a duty to review terminology for potential stereotypical bias in this field. Trauma is regarded as an emotional reaction based upon an inner working framework which was created in a context of adverse childhood experiences. The foundation of a pedagogy and the message which is given to service-users is hope and potential for change. For example, the Scottish Family Support Strategy, 2020–2023, uses the voice, validation and hope model (Glasgow City Council, 2020). This model promotes that practitioners and families discuss issues as unresolved trauma, which implies potential for positive change, as opposed to unresolved parents, which imposes a negative status upon the parent's identity.

Unresolved trauma can only be resolved if the parent is supported to develop his or her sense of self and agency and to take ownership of the child's destiny. I practise in a multigenerational context, and I have found that longevity of change and minimisation of intergenerational transmission of trauma can be achieved. Children, parents, and grandparents learn to work alongside the professional and together as a family unit. Families who use drugs or alcohol can improve their lifestyles over time, but there are always peaks and troughs in the change processes. A wide network of available supportive adults, out-with the immediate family, can also provide multiple protective factors.

The second and third trimester of pregnancy are often opportune times to implement intervention. These stages naturally incur the mother developing maternal representation of her unborn baby. This maternal comprehension of the forthcoming baby informs the mother's inner working model. The working model of the child interview (Theran et al., 2005) can be used to categorise the mother's representation of the forthcoming baby as balanced, disengaged, or distorted. Negative childhood experiences may result in inadequate parenting if a pregnant woman develops a disengaged or a distorted mental representation of her unborn baby. I have recently learned that fathers experience physical changes during pregnancy, which includes an increase in cortisol levels in the early stages and a reduction in the production of testosterone pre-birth. Physical changes for both parents occur in tandem with emotional and mental representations of their unborn baby emerging.

Belsky (1984) described three determinants of parenting as the personal psychological resources of parents, the characteristics of the child, and the contextual sources of stress and support. Contextual sources which Belsky regarded as inducing stress, or giving support were marital relationship, social networks, and employment. The research by this author identified that personal resources of the parent were more effective in enhancing the parent–child relationship than contextual sources of support. Additionally, contextual sources had a greater impact upon the parent–child relationship than the characteristics of the child.

The literature review by O'Hara et al. (2019) accessed 22 publications on parent–child and family–child interventions to examine the impact of video feedback upon parental sensitivity. The studies were conducted in Canada, the Netherlands, the United Kingdom, and the United States of America. Single studies were also conducted in Italy, Germany, Lithuania, Norway, and Portugal. Findings indicated that the sensitivity of parents did increase with the use of feedback from videos of parent–child interactions. Visual media are excellent tools to use in parenting work and encompass photographs, videos, narratives, or role-play. It is important that parents are supported to interpret a photograph or video and to link their increase in comprehension to development of skills.

Box 4.2 Example from practice

Jenny and her mother, Nikki, were referred to our service by social worker and health workers. The referral identified generic parenting work as a useful approach to increase attachment between mother and child. This intervention took the format of four stay-and-play sessions which I facilitated through presentation of specific toys and by guiding the parent in reacting and interacting with her young daughter during the session. Jenny was 30 months old.

At an initial parenting session, I always set out a selection of toys which can provide opportunities for exploration and development in each area of growth, and the process of play exhibits the way in which mother and daughter relate to one another. Additionally, the interactions express the interests and needs of Jenny and her stage of development. All of this information gives me guidance on setting up an appropriate environment for week two, and beyond.

Jenny and her mother entered the small therapeutic room. The blue roller blinds had been lowered to minimise distraction from the wet and windy weather and to direct Jenny's attention to the activities. A tall corner light shone down upon the scene, highlighting a rich learning environment. I had put pastel-coloured yoga mats upon the floor and a small selection of toys, some tucked safely inside long-life bags and other items displayed attractively in situ to invite investigation and creativity. The little girl immediately sat down to study a jigsaw.

As Jenny was discovering how to remove each animal piece by shaking the board, I took the opportunity to offer Nikki the choice of a folder from several options. Nikki quickly declared that purple was her favourite colour. I handed the young mum a marker pen to write her name and to take ownership of this aspect of the intervention. I explained that the play sessions would involve interactions with Jenny and Nikki. I would sit aside from the yoga mats unless Jenny invited me into the domain of her mother and self. I would use questions, prompts, and make suggestions during play to extend Jenny's learning and enrich the interactions. Together, we would decide which parts of the play to photograph, and these memories would rapidly fill the purple folder, accompanied by Nikki's responses and action points. As I struggled to use the digital camera, Nikki leant forward spontaneously, and she guided me competently and confidently in mastering the digital media. These little spontaneous actions are consequential and contribute to an effective practitioner–parent dyad.

Week by week, I met with Nikki and noticed her gaining self-esteem. Many brightly coloured photographs quickly filled the pages of Nikki's folder and included her interpretation and understanding on the importance of play, attachment, and good physical and mental health. I sat next to this young mother as she opened the folder depicting interactions from the previous week. Nikki always smiled shyly as she viewed the mother and child play scenes, and she looked at me expectantly.

Taking time to give parents an awareness of their skills is invaluable to parenting work and creates a strong, positive foundation of hope for change. I pointed to the details within each photograph and commented upon Nikki's open body language, her broad smile, eye contact with her little girl, the use of gestures to indicate questions, the offering of two choices for boundary setting, one toy in each hand, just out of reach to encourage thinking time for Jenny. I drew an imaginary triangle on one photograph: Nikki, Jenny, and the toys. I indicated an elastic thread from Nikki to Jenny and stretching beyond towards the activities as the child had gained confidence in exploring out of physical touch of her mother's circle of security. I turned a page quickly to access a special photograph and to remind Nikki of the enormous bear hug which she had given to Jenny at the end of session one.

We talked about aspects of good physical health and mental health, and jointly we created our definition of attachment. We considered sleep and food as contributory aspects of a learning journey, and we agreed that family life has good moments and many challenging times. We explored and interpreted the communication methods of Jenny into questions, insecurities, needs, wants and interests: her high-pitched screams and throwing toys, hitting her mother, and spitting on the furniture. We identified and captured Jenny's fleeting eye contact, her gentle touches, the golden smile that slowly spread across her face, and her excited happy body language as she jumped, and jumped, and jumped again. We understood the world of Jenny, and we gained insight into this little girl's quest for her mother's attention, positive or negative. Together, we considered approaches to promoting positive behaviour in a context of learning and not reprimanding. Nikki gained confidence as I expressed, "there's a solution for everything … what do *you* think?"

Home and services

Media, in the form of photographs or videos, has transformed parenting work over the past 40 years of my career. In general, parents are enlightened by reviewing their parenting strategies, recognising inherent skills, and creating different approaches with the support and guidance of a practitioner. It is an exciting and fulfilling pathway for an early years practitioner to take alongside a parent. Change takes time, it is challenging, there are peaks and troughs and plateau periods in which development of parent and child appears to be stationary. As practitioners, we contribute to a lifelong learning journey for parent and child; we provide memories full of knowledge and understanding that may remain latent for many years but can be activated for use in the right conditions. Small impacts have great potential for development of human beings.

The COVID-19 pandemic is a current adversity which to date appears to impose long-term impact upon mental health, and one significant area is loneliness through isolation periods of lockdown within many countries. The importance of self has been highlighted to the public and governments across the world throughout 2020–2022, and the topic is a current area of research (Moore & Churchill, 2020). Twenty years ago, Trevarthen (2001) published findings upon companionship and infant mental health. This researcher identified collaborative intersubjectivity as significant for good mental health and brain development in the early years, and impactful upon interpersonal needs through the entire lifespan. Babies have been shown to participate in reciprocal interactions at 6 weeks of age that are accompanied by emotional expressions.

A play environment is a useful context in which to commence this process. The infant's resilience to positive stresses from low-level negative influences is nurtured and promoted during interactions with peers. This experience forms an excellent foundation for gaining resilience to toxic stress. Resilience is incremental and created over a period of time. Personality, family circumstances and outlook on life, and the extended social support system are factors that affect the child's resilience.

Current thinking indicates that demonstration of cognitive ability can change over time, and the processes are affected by external and internal factors relating to proximal and distal supports, or childhood adversities. Neural circuits may respond rapidly to maturation in the period from birth to three years. Alternatively, circuits relating to executive functioning continue to be sensitive to influences throughout childhood *and* adulthood (Boyce et al. 2021). Childhood adversities may impose effects from latent influences many years after the adverse event has occurred (Whitters, 2020); however, maternal responsivity in the adolescent years can reduce negative impacts (Boyce et al. 2021). Changing the operational skills of an individual is best achieved through intervention with the extended family unit. Families require sensitive, responsive support, and guidance in rethinking interpretation of their world, and subsequently the chemical reactions in the body will change and toxic stress reactions will reduce for individuals and future generations.

The recent findings of Boyce et al. (2021) referred to individual susceptibility to adversity and links between unsupportive parenting and increased inflammatory reactions throughout the lifespan, particularly in a context of significant life events. Resilience is adaptation to adversity that reduces the negative impact upon learning and well-being. Research has indicated the significance of a mother–infant communication to secure attachment which contributes to appropriate conditions for adaptation (Beebe & Steele, 2013; Zeanah et al., 1994). Alongside targeted and specific intervention for families is daily universal support from early years settings which is implemented by practitioners who are trained in trauma-informed practice. Timing an intervention to a pre-crisis context is dependent on services working collaboratively by sharing information on concerns and by ensuring that families are supported to express their needs and anxieties.

McCrory et al. (2017) conducted a study that underlined the significance of preventative intervention. Findings indicated that maltreatment could cause alteration in neural networks and cognition, which resulted in latent vulnerability to developing a psychiatric disorder in later life. The six core strengths to minimise violent tendencies can be nurtured from birth (Perry et al., 1995). This research team applied the terms of attachment, self-regulation, affiliation, attunement, tolerance, and respect as representative of these strengths. A child who expresses an act of violence may give justification in relation to his current cognitive interpretation of the world, but the violent tendency is actually based upon emotions which are stored in the limbic system, created during his earliest experiences of life (Perry et al., 1995).

The two systems for responding to stress are the sympathomedullary (SAM) system, and the hypothalmic-pituitary-adrenal axis. It was useful for my own practice to learn that the hormone adrenalin, as a regulator of cell or organ activity, can take up to 20 minutes to course around the body through the bloodstream. An emergency universal energy store of adenosine triphosphate (ATP) is situated within muscles to enable an immediate response. Chemical energy is released which triggers a physical reaction to threat based upon survival strategies. The external stress results in internal changes as epinephrine (adrenalin) increases circulation and breathing rates and releases glycogen throughout the body. The body makes this response based upon rapid assessment of an immediate threat.

I consider these findings in the context of my practice within the birth to 2-year-old playroom. Referrals for placements in the service give details of perceived stresses upon babies and children, for example, domestic violence, drug use, parents' additional support needs, and mental-health issues. Additional underlying factors to vulnerability include poverty, seeking asylum, community violence, and isolation. At entry to the service, I observe that many children are vigilant, which is demonstrated by quick reactions and physical withdrawal from assumed sources of threat: adults or peers breaching the infant's safety space around the body, unexpected movements in the visual peripheries, and loud indeterminate noises from outside the vicinity. Physical and emotional contact is immediately given to the infant who demonstrates rapid heartbeat and perspiration. Nurturing and reassurance are offered to the infant but may be rejected in the early stages of a relationship and interpreted as potential threat. Responses can appear as an overreaction by an infant to local issues, and it is essential that practitioners appreciate the ongoing impact of current or historical adversities from out-with the setting.

An understanding can be gained of the complex internal working of an infant in this context and the potential exhaustion which the body and mind experience during and after these episodes. The practitioner presents a buffering relationship to minimise the effects but equally importantly by offering positive experiences within the child's world to reconfigure his inner working model and to use the secure attachment relationship for the optimum outcomes. Babies require time to assimilate the positive relationship overtures and to adjust internally which can be observed in external behaviour. The skill of observation in services is key to understanding mental health in infants, and adults, and providing responsive care for the individual.

The hormone cortisol has positive effects in the short-term timescale and negative effects in long-term periods as stress is prolonged. The circadian rhythm as the 24-hour cycle of light and dark regulates cortisol levels; however, lifestyles can cause changes to these patterns. Many families that our service supports do not adhere to the traditional pattern of sleep during darkness and activity during daylight hours. Parents can spend hours on internet activity during the night and struggle to cope with a waking baby in the early hours of sunrise. Long-term stress results in lengthy periods in which the body experiences high levels of cortisol which impacts adversely upon cognitive skill, blood sugar, blood pressure, and ability to sleep.

The knowledge of the destructive properties of cortisol provides rationale to strategic planning and funding for intervention (National Scientific Council on the Developing Child, 2006). In addition, I feel that practice is greatly informed through understanding that excessive cortisol can stop neural connections occurring and create stress reactions which are barriers to learning and achievement of potential. A baby's lifestyle is profoundly disrupted if the primary carer's parenting skills are affected by toxic stress. In turn, the baby experiences this toxic stress albeit indirectly from the source that affects his parents. During these episodes, the baby's hippocampus, which is the area of the limbic system that supports memory and links to emotion and sensory learning, produces less cortisol receptors. Stress remains at a high level.

High levels of stress can also result in the stress response system being *underactive*. I have frequently observed the practical presentation of babies and young children, who operate within a lifestyle of stress factors, as being non-responsive and challenging to stimulate with learning opportunities. The baby has learned to minimise the potential for stress to occur by limiting any interactions with adults, despite the context of a nurturing nursery. These effects represent primitive dissociative adaptations and physical or cognitive freeze. Dissociation is accompanied by a physiological response to prepare the body and mind for reducing the effect of threat: the heart rate slows down, blood may flow away from extremities, endogenous opioids reduce physical pain and flood the mind with a sensation of calmness and psychological distancing from attack.

In the early stages of my career, the children who presented with these characteristics were termed still children which depicted their body language. During the 1980s and 1990s, we recorded this behaviour and devised practical strategies to support re-engagement. As early years practitioners, we did not have access to scientific knowledge or comprehension from research. As a professional, I have always sought understanding of my work; however, I can recall supporting these still children without the benefit of theory and understanding. In Scotland, it is only since professional registration was introduced that practitioners can access research databases through NHS sites (Scottish Social Services Council, 2003). Research has enriched the role of the early years workforce. Completing postgraduate study over the past 20 years, and professional registration that incurs continuous development, have given me opportunities to fulfil my desire for knowledge by reference to current research and theory.

The drive to achieve perfection can have positive or negative effects upon the child's well-being and his involvement with learning. Many high-level intellectual or creative outcomes can be achieved which are based upon the child's rationale of a perfect goal; however, a child may never be satisfied with his own work. Consistent use of positive praise by primary carers may actually hinder his intrinsic motivation. Interpretation of the world at heightened sensitivity, physically or emotionally, can lead to a child experiencing a sense of failure and an unusually negative reaction if outcomes are not achieved.

Almost 40 years ago, Roedell (1984) conducted research that explored the emotional status of children with high ability and focused upon their vulnerabilities. Findings indicated correlation between an increasing level of advancement and a risk of the child exhibiting social maladjustment. Roedell highlighted a lack of confidence as the prevailing sign of maladjustment in this research study. Contexts were identified as a tendency to seek perfectionism, high adult expectations of the child's output, an increase in emotional and physical sensitivity, and, interestingly, role conflicts. The latter refers to the child's immature sense of self and dependency on extrinsic motivation from primary carers.

Role conflict can occur in a context of family, community, or societal expectations of a child which are often based upon socio-economic circumstances, culture, or gender. Chichekian and Shore (2014) placed importance upon the influence of social interaction on learning, but children may lack confidence or skill in seeking assistance from others. Some children may demonstrate preference for solitary or parallel play and actively reject opportunities for cooperative constructive play.

Children quickly adopt the social code of a service or family and understand an implicit child-imposed ranking system that can denote acceptance or rejection in the group and subsequently promote an increase or decrease in self-confidence. Zhou and Brown (2015) suggested that self-appointed ranking can also adversely affect a child's sense of efficacy.

Environment provides a rich learning arena that immerses a child in his family influences, in addition to the local community and national culture. Vygotsky (1994) highlights the influences from a changing environment, which may incur circumstantial adaptation of the context, and, consequently, the child's increase or decrease in involvement within this arena. It seems that an environment instigates change in the child which is prompted by his evolving interactions with learning opportunities. The learner's interpretation of and reaction to an environment alters as he assimilates knowledge, gains understanding, and reconfigures his inner working model (Bowlby, 1979). This adapted inner working model inevitably affects his actions and emotions. Tronick and Beeghly (2011) described the outcome as a new bio-psychosocial state of consciousness within the child.

Tronick and Beeghly (2011) conducted research on the ways in which infants acquire meaning and explored the issue within a context of mental health in young children. The adult–child dyad is regarded as integral to a child's capacity to learn. The positive reciprocal relationships with adults create a foundation for a child to potentially achieve the zone of proximal development. This system enables scaffolding of knowledge from adult to child which is responsive to individual needs, interests, and well-being at any moment in time. The adult–child system also promotes the child's self-regulation of emotions by presenting opportunities to copy reactions and to adopt coping mechanisms within the daily learning context.

Involvement underpins the mesosystem which links home and services by practitioner, parent, and child sharing a positive attitude towards learning opportunities. El Nokali et al. (2010) describe one measure of parental involvement in an education system as quality and frequency of communication with teaching staff. These authors indicated that this involvement may be considered as a static predictor of positive outcomes within the context of schooling. It was concluded that this is an aspect that contributes to an increase in motivation for learning in children and young people. Some years later, a study by Weiss (2019) also found that behaviours associated with learning, for example motivation and persistence, were variables that could be used to predict future academic success in formal schooling: high scores in reading and writing were associated in the research with parental involvement in learning within a home environment.

References

Asmussen, K., Fischer, F., Drayton, E., & McBride, T. (2020). Adverse childhood experiences, what we know, what we don't know, and what should happen next. https://www.eif.org.uk/report/adverse-childhood-experiences-what-we-know-what-we-dont-know-and-what-should-happen-next.

Association of Infant Mental Health United Kingdom. (2021). The secondary impact of COVID-19 on infant mental health: What do we know, and what digital methods of working can improve outcomes. AIMHUK best practice guide number 8. https://aimh.uk/news-resources/members-only-resources.

Beebe B., & Steele, M. (2013). How does microanalysis of mother–infant communication inform maternal sensitivity and infant attachment? *Attachment & Human Development* 15(5–6),583–602.

Belsky, J. (1984). The determinants of parenting: A process model. *Child Development*, 55(*1*), 83–96. https://doi.org/10.2307/1129836.

Bowlby, J. (1979). *The making and breaking of affectional bonds*. Abingdon and New York: Routledge.

Boyce, W. T., Levitt, P., Martinez, F. D., McEwen, B. S., & Shonkoff, J. P. (2021). Genes, environments, and time: The biology of adversity and resilience. *Pediatrics*, 147(2), e20201651. https://doi.org/10.1542/peds.2020-1651.

Bratton, S. C., Landreth, G. L., Kellam, T., & Blackard, S. R. (2006). *Child/parent participation therapy treatment manual*. Abingdon and New York: Routledge.

Bronfenbrenner, U. (1979). *The ecology of human development*, 2nd edition. Cambridge, MA: Harvard University Press.

Chichekian, T., & Shore, B. M. (2014). The international baccalaureate: Contributing to the use of inquiry in higher education teaching and learning. In J. M. Carfora & P. Blessinger (Eds.), *Inquiry-based learning for faculty and institutional development: A conceptual and practical resource for educators*, vol. I (pp. 73–97). Bingley: Emerald Group.

Choi, J., Jeong, B., Rohan, M. L., & Polcari, A. (2008). Preliminary evidence for white matter tract abnormalities in young adults exposed to parental verbal abuse. *Biological Psychiatry*, 65(3), 227–234.

Cicchetti, D., & Toth, S. L. (2006). Developmental psychopathology and preventive intervention. In W. Damon & R. Lerner (Eds.), *Handbook of child psychology*, vol. IV (pp. 511–512). Hoboken, NJ: John Wiley & Sons.

Coates, D. (2010). Impact of childhood abuse: Biopsychosocial pathways through which adult mental health is compromised article in Australian social work. *Australian Social Work*, 63(4), 391–403.

Doidge, N. (2008). *The brain that changes itself.* New York: Penguin.

El Nokali, N. E., Bachman, H. J., & Votruba-Drzal, E. (2010). Parent involvement and children's academic and social development in elementary school. *Child Development*, 81(3), 988–1005.

Fonagy, P. (1999). Pathological attachments and therapeutic action. *Psyche Matters.* https://www.psychematters.com/papers/fonagy3.htm.

Fraiberg, S., Adelson, E., & Shapiro, V. (1975) Ghosts in the nursery: A psychoanalytic approach to the problems of impaired infant-mother relationships. *Journal of American Academy for Child Development*, 14(3), 387–421. https://www.sciencedirect.com/science/article/pii/S0002713809614424.

Glasgow City Council. (2020). *Glasgow's family support Strategy, 2020–23.* https://www.glasgow.gov.uk/councillorsandcommittees/viewSelectedDocument.asp?c=P62AFQDN0GUTT181DX.

Gunnar, M. R., & Barr, R. G. (1998). Stress, early brain development, and behavior. *Infants and Young Children*, 11(1), 1–14. https://journals.lww.com/iycjournal/Abstract/1998/07000/Stress_Early_Brain_Development_and_Behaviour.4.aspx.

National Scientific Council on the Developing Child. (2020). Connecting the brain to the rest of the body: Early childhood development and lifelong health are deeply intertwined. Working paper no. 15. https://www.developingchild.harvard.edu.

Hetherington, K. (2020). *Ending childhood adversity: A public health approach.* Edinburgh: Public Health Scotland.

McClelland, J. L. (1998). Complementary learning systems in the brain: A connectionist approach to explicit and implicit cognition and memory. *Annals of the New York Academy of Sciences*, 153–178. https://www.semanticscholar.org/paper/Complementary-Learning-Systems-in-the-Brain%3A-A-to-McClelland/67d91b41134fd099f962568d77abe235582748ab.

McCrory, E. J., Gerin, M. I., & Viding, E. (2017). Childhood maltreatment, latent vulnerability and the shift to preventative psychiatry: The contribution of functional brain imaging. *Annual Research Review.* https://doi.org/10.1111/jcpp.12713.

Milot, T., St-Laurent, D., & Ethier, L. S. (2016). Intervening with severely and chronically neglected children and their families: The contribution of trauma-informed approaches. *Child Abuse Review*, 25, 89–101.

Moore, E., & Churchill, G. (2020). Still here for children: Sharing the experiences of NSPCC staff who supported children and families during the Covid-2019 pandemic.

https://learning.nspcc.org.uk/research-resources/2020/still-here-for-children-experiences-of-nspcc-staff-during-coronavirus.

National Scientific Council on the Developing Child. (2006). Early exposure to toxic substances damages brain architecture. Working paper no. 4. https://developingchild.harvard.edu/resources/early-exposure-to-toxic-substances-damages-brain-architecture.

O'Hara, L., Smith, E. R., Barlow, J., Livingstone, N., Herath, N. I. N. S., Wei, Y., Spreckelsen, T., & Macdonald, G. (2019). Video feedback for parental sensitivity and attachment security in children under five years. *Cochrane Database of Systematic Reviews*, (11). https://www.cochrane.org/CD012348/BEHAV_video-feedback-parental-sensitivity-and-child-attachment.

Perry, B. D., Pollard, R., Blakely, T., Baker, W., & Vigilante, D. (1995). Childhood trauma, the neurobiology of the brain: How "states" become "traits". *Infant Mental Health Journal*, 16(4), 271–291.

Roedell, W. C. (1984). Vulnerabilities of highly gifted children. *Roeper Review* 6(*3*), 127–130. https://www.positivedisintegration.com/Roedell1984.

Rogers, C. (1990). Toward a modern approach to values: The valuing process in the mature person. In H. Kirschenbaum & V. L. Henderson (Eds.), *The Carl Rogers Reader*. London: Constable.

Roisman, G. I., Padron, E., Sroufe, A., & Egeland, B. (2003). Earned–secure attachment status in retrospect and prospect. *Child Development*. 73(4), 1204–1219. https://www.srcd.onlinelibrary.wiley.com/doi/abs/10.1111/1467-8624.00467.

Rothschild, B. (2000). *The body remembers: The psychophysiology of trauma and trauma treatment*. London: W. W. Norton & Company.

Schechter, D., Wilheim, E., Suardi, F., & Serpa, S. R. (2019). The effects of violent experiences on infants and young children. In C. H. Zeanah, Jr (Ed.), *Handbook of infant mental health*, 4th edition (pp. 219–238). New York: The Guilford Press.

Schore, A. N. (1994). *Affect regulation and the origin of self: The neurobiology of emotional development*. Hillsdale, NJ: Erlbaum.

Scottish Government. (2004). *A curriculum for excellence*. Edinburgh: Scottish Executive.

Scottish Government & NHS Scotland. (2021). Trauma-informed practice: A toolkit for Scotland. https://www.gov.scot/publications/trauma-informed-practice-toolkit-scotland.

Scottish Social Services Council. (2003). *Codes of practice for social services workers and employers, code 1*. Dundee: Scottish Social Services Council.

Shonkoff, J. P., Boyce, W. T., Levitt, P., & Fernando, D. (2021). Leveraging the biology of adversity and resilience to transform pediatric practice. *Pediatrics*, 147(2), 1–9.

Siegel, D. J. (2003). An interpersonal neurobiology of psychotherapy: The developing mind and the resolution of trauma. In M. F. Solomon & D. J. Siegel (Eds.), *Healing trauma, attachment, mind, body, and brain* (pp. 1–56). London: W. W. Norton & Company.

Teicher, M. T., Andersen, S. L., Polcari, A., Andersen, C. M., Navalta, C. P. (2002). Developmental neurobiology of childhood stress and trauma. *Review Psychiatry*, 25 (2), 397–426. https://www.pubmed.ncbi.nlm.nih.gov/12136507.

Teicher, M. H., Dumont, N. L., Yutaka, I., Vaituzis, C., Giedd, J. N., & Andersen, L. (2004). Childhood neglect is associated with reduced corpus callosum area. *Journal of Biopsychiatry*, 56(2), 80–85. https://www.pubmed.ncbi.nlm.nih.gov/?term=teicher+mh&cauthor_id=15231439.

The Family Nurse Partnership (2011). The evaluation of the Family Nurse Partnership programme in Scotland: Phase 1 report – intake and early pregnancy. https://www.gov.scot/publications/evaluation-family-nurse-partnership-programme-scotland-phase-1-report-intake-early-pregnancy.

Theran, S., Levendosky, A., Bogat, G., & Huth-Bocks, A. (2005). Stability and change in mothers' internal representations of their infants over time. *Attachment & Human Development*, 7(3), 253–268. https://www.tandfonline.com/doi/abs/10.1080/14616730500245609.

Trevarthen, C. (2001). Intrinsic motives for companionship in understanding: Their origin, development, and significance for infant mental health. *Infant Mental Health Journal*, 22 (1–2),95–131. https://www.researchgate.net/publication/247947166_Intrinsic_motives.

Tronick, E., & Beeghly, M. (2011). Infants' meaning-making and the development of mental health problems. *American Psychologist*, 66(2), 107–109. https://www.pubmed.ncbi.nlm.nih.gov/21142336.

Vygotsky, L. S. (1978). *Mind in society: The development of higher psychological processes*. Cambridge, MA: Harvard University Press.

Vygotsky, L. S. (1994). The problem of the cultural development of the child. In R. Van der Veer & J. Valsiner (Eds.), *The Vygotsky reader* (pp. 57–71, 308–310). Oxford: Blackwell.

Weiss, L. (2019). Wechsler intelligence scale for children, fifth edition: Use in societal context. In L. G. Weiss, D. H. Saklofske, J. A. Holdnack, & A. Prifitera (Eds.), *Practical resources for the mental health professional*, 2nd edition (pp. 129–195). Academic Press.

Whitters, H. G. (2019). *Attainment and executive functioning in the early years: Research for inclusive practice and lifelong learning*. Abingdon and New York: Routledge.

Whitters, H. G. (2020). *Adverse childhood experiences, attachment, and the early years learning environment*. Abingdon and New York: Routledge.

Zeanah, C. H., Benoit, D., Hirshberg, L., Barton, M. L., & Regan, C. (1994). Mothers' representations of their infants are concordant with infant attachment classifications. *Developmental Issues in Psychiatry and Psychology*, 1, 9–18. http://www.researchgate.net/publications/285330060.

Zhou, M., & Brown, D. (2015). *Educational learning theories*, 2nd edition, Education Open Textbooks, 1. https://oer.galileo.usg.edu/education-textbooks/1.

5 Ability, capacity, and creativity

This chapter presents teaching and learning as interdependent partners that blend within a symbiotic relationship. Teaching should capitalise upon the child's initial level of understanding, and incrementally support and influence realisation of potential for children of all abilities. The research by Roedell (1984) on significant uneven development in young children who had higher than average ability is presented. The recommendations by Fidler (2006) on promoting a child's developmental strengths are discussed in relation to additional learning needs.

Four levels of intervention are described within the play cycle (King & Sturrock, 2020), and organisation of neural networks is contextualised as time-dependent or experience-dependent. Perry (1997) related disruptions to a lack of sensory experiences during critical periods of development or the direct impact of adversities upon the infant. Attention restoration theory (Ohly et al., 2016) is accessed to explain an increase in and restoration of executive functioning through exposure to natural environments. Exemplars are given to represent hard and soft fascination activities. Csikszentmihalyi et al. (2018) emphasised the complexity of the psychological aspects of flow theory and the systems model of creativity is used to increase knowledge and understanding of links between capacity, creativity, and emotional well-being.

Teaching and learning

Some years ago, I was collecting data by observing participants who were children aged 4–5 years and teachers within a context of early years in primary schools. I noted that several teachers were so busy teaching a planned lesson to a class that they did not notice, or respond spontaneously, to the children learning. Delivery of the lessons was constricted by curricular expectations, professional accountability, and restrictive timetables based upon predicted attainment. These circumstances bypass the use of scaffolding and sensitive responding and decrease the opportunities for creative and imaginative ideas to be fulfilled. Potential to reach a higher level of learning is reduced.

Teaching should always encompass periods in which an educator is informed by observing and by understanding each child's learning processes

DOI: 10.4324/9781003358107-5

as he interacts with an environment and peers. Observations of children should facilitate identification of the aptitudes of individual pupils and record the changing of abilities over time. Observations should also recognise pupil motivation and application to overcome obstacles in completing tasks. Snapshot or planned observations, even for a few minutes, can be rich sources of understanding of a child's ability, capacity, and motivation to learn.

Teaching and learning are interdependent partners, and each process directly impacts upon the other. The creation of a lesson plan, or a nursery activity, is a preparatory stage of the learning process within an educator-to-child relationship. The plan may only have momentary value as a child's reaction and response to this knowledge exchange commences an iterative reciprocal process between adult and child. Consequently, the plan should be adaptable and responsive to the child's capacity and ability to learn. Teaching and learning are merged within a symbiotic relationship. Delivery of knowledge should be shaped and led by activation of a child's learning processes. Teaching should capitalise upon the child's initial level of understanding and incrementally support and influence realisation of potential for children of all abilities.

Blumenfeld et al. (2006) noted that an effective learning environment depended upon knowledge of a teacher, knowledge and experience of a learner, design of tasks, and community influences. These authors reported that outcomes of a learning environment should relate to learning in academic, social, metacognitive, and developmental categories. In early years practice, learning encompasses all these outcomes, and broad holistic opportunities are key aspects in implementation of a curriculum in the child's earliest years. Multimodal environments provide children with a range of learning materials and a range of media in which to demonstrate achievement. A rich environment responds to children's interests, needs, and wishes, in addition to reflecting a curriculum.

Siegel (2003) discusses complexity of neural processes as the result of differentiation and integration. Opportunities to achieve this optimum state occur within stimulating environments, and good mental health is the self-organisational process that supports this system. Exposure to experiences leads to neural firing patterns. Siegel estimated that there are millions of firing patterns within a human brain.

Memory

Memory is formed through integration that inputs to a holistic information system. It is known that during rapid eye movement sleep experiences are associated with consolidation and integration of emotions and knowledge (Siegel, 2003).

Explicit memory has two forms: semantic or factual memory and episodic or autobiographical memory. Autobiographical memory includes a sense of self in the memory recall and an awareness of time. There are two known components to implicit memory: procedural memory, which is associated with behaviour, and the emotions accompanying an experience. For example, the actions required to ride a bike are retained in procedural memory, and the associated emotion which may be positive or negative remain within implicit memory. Siegel (2003) makes an interesting point as he described the potential for an implicit memory in the earliest years being retained as a *sense* of familiarity as opposed to actual remembering of details. Young children may recall and express emotions and reactions to experiences that occurred before effective communication skills had been established. This recall is based upon the sense of familiarity.

It is fascinating that the brain has the ability to process past experiences at a higher level over time as development and maturity occur. This creates rationale for the use of counselling in adulthood which targets unresolved trauma from childhood. Hart and Rubia (2012) highlighted the impact of childhood maltreatment upon brain architecture and functions. Adversity in childhood impacts upon infant mental health. The infant experiences internal issues, for example, anxiety, and demonstrates external behaviours, for example, poor impulse control. Long-term changes to the infant's brain architecture and functioning can occur. These authors indicated links between child abuse and deficits in intellect, memory, working memory, attention, response inhibition, and the ability to discriminate between emotions.

The therapeutic process provides verbal media to support resolution of trauma by enabling an individual to create a coherent narrative of the issues. Additionally, this process provides non-verbal media in the form of a secure attachment relationship that supports self-regulation and integration of experiences. Lack of resolution of trauma is regarded as the mind's incapacity to balance differentiation and integration of energy and information flow (Siegel, 2003).

Stress interferes with integration and differentiation, but a therapeutic relationship can fulfil the purpose of liberating the mind from these barriers and by supporting a desire to achieve maximum complexity. Siegel (2003) studied the mind and brain, and this researcher concluded that the mind emerges as the brain matures. The development of the mind is influenced by self, and others, and affected by personality. Interaction occurs between neurophysiological and interpersonal relationships. Over time, neural connections can be made independently and separate from the influences of the therapeutic dyad. Sensory input, for example, auditory, visual, or tactile, can affect perceptions and direct actions. These processes are often associated with creativity.

Differentiation is influenced by genetics and experiences, particularly during the earliest years. It is the young child's involvement with learning experiences that is key to development, and not solely the environment per se. It is essential that practitioners and parents appreciate and embrace the value of their role in supporting a child's engagement, interaction, and response to learning.

Siegel (2003) clarified internal and external constraints, and this author identified self-regulation as essential to good mental health. Internal constraints refer to the composition of synaptic connections among neurons. External constraints refer to environmental experiences and include interpersonal communication with others, particularly if a relationship has an emotional significance. A relationship is an external factor that can influence the neural system by leading to changes in internal constraints. Positive changes increase the potential for complexity to be achieved.

Secure attachment is a descriptor of the relationship which a child has created with another person, for example, a parent, carer, peer, or practitioner. The child may have different types of relationships with his range of carers. Fosha (2003) identified skills which are required by a caregiver to nurture a secure attachment status with a child, and to achieve optimal development. These skills or characteristics apply to parents and practitioners in early years settings.

- Adult's affective competence.
- Adult's reflective self-function.
- Adult's capacity to support periods of repair following short-term rupture of the relationship.

Therapeutic intervention can support neural integration between the right and left hemisphere of the brain and impact positively upon the effects of unresolved trauma. The term "earned–secure" was used by Roisman et al. (2002) in relation to an adult who has achieved secure attachment within her relationships despite a history of negative relational experiences. A 23-year-longitudinal study was conducted with adult participants who had insecure attachments in childhood. Findings indicated that a change in relationship potential impacted favourably upon secure attachments between the participants and their children.

High ability

It has been recognised for many years that identification of children who are developmentally delayed is an important consideration in implementing early intervention (Pfeiffer & Petscher, 2008). However, children of high ability should also be identified and supported in response to individual learning needs.

A study by Freeman (1998) was conducted over twenty years ago, and the knowledge and understanding from findings continues to be applied by current educators. Recommendations were compiled into guidance for teachers regarding recognition of pupils who had high ability. Freeman focused mainly on assessment of teacher–pupil interaction in a school setting. Findings included checklists that contained ability criteria, for example, the use of complicated rules and extensive imaginative play, alacrity in the use of symbolic communication – talking, reading, and writing – and extended concentration on tasks from an early age. The conclusion of this research highlighted circumstances that accompanied problem-solving and a child's ability to respond to unexpected circumstances within a learning context as significant factors.

There are points found on many checklists that provide a useful foundation for learning about universal traits associated with ability. Examples are memory and retention of factual knowledge, regulation of oneself, and identification of preference for learning style and medium. Freeman's research indicates that the use of checklists can provide knowledge to an educator and promote professional awareness of the concept of ability, but the author warns that checklists can be self-limiting (Freeman, 1998). Mental health is currently regarded as influential to the learning context. This aspect does not specifically feature on Freeman's guide to educators.

Intelligence is understood by Freeman (1998) as a way of organising and using knowledge in relation to a physical and social environment. Findings did refer to the influence from culture and family upon development, and the study concluded that every child's potential can be realised with encouragement, learning materials, and educational support. Freeman's study outlined the use of two intelligence quotient (IQ) tests to determine ability in a context of chronological age. Findings indicated that testing was applicable to measuring a child's academic ability within the early years of a school environment.

- Stanford-Binet test is based upon verbal interaction.
- Wechsler Intelligence Scales are based upon mathematics.

Wechsler was an American psychologist who used statistical standardisation to determine the ranking of an individual in relation to the norms of the general population within a particular age-range. Wechsler created a standard IQ of mean = 100, and standard deviation = 15, and he applied this approach to different tests. The Wechsler scale for young children was established in 2004, in France, and termed WPPSI-111 (Vaivre-Douret, 2011). This scale can be used to measure IQ of children aged from 2 years and 6 months until 7 years and 4 months.

The indicators by Freeman (1998) are still applicable today and provide support to educators in understanding the capacity and ability of all children to learn. A few years ago, Renzulli grouped ability under three clusters as a means of identification in order to provide education which nurtured academic, and creative achievement (Renzulli, 2019). This educator applied the term three-ring conception of giftedness to represent three aspects.

1   Ability which is greater than the norm for a child's age group.
2   Task commitment.
3   Creativity.

Forty years ago, Renzulli (1978) conducted research that indicated that the aforementioned three clusters of ability, task commitment, and creativity were equal partners in contributing to a child's overall ability. Recent research by Renzulli and Reis (2018) concluded that gifted behaviour is reflected by interaction of these three clusters which could be applied to any area of human development. The researchers emphasised that the three clusters did not need to be present for a child to exhibit high ability. The constant factor was demonstration of interaction by two or more clusters at a higher level than the norm. Findings indicated that task commitment and creativity tend to be applied together.

It is enlightening to consider research that investigates issues beyond the immediate scope of a research topic. As a researcher and practitioner in early years, my focus for this monograph is infant mental health; however, the discussion by Renzulli and Reis (2018), albeit in relation to high ability, certainly contributes to understanding of generic learning processes. In addition, I refer to research in children who have additional support for learning needs. Understanding of the norm can be strengthened by information on outliers.

Ability

Ability is multilayered, and initial subdivisions relate to the use of cognitive and physical skill that demonstrate the child's level of prowess. Physical skill can be further refined by consideration of fine and gross motor skills, spatial awareness, and proprioception. Ability can be extended through copying which encompasses a child's interpretation and reproduction of what he has observed, including elements of creativity. The skill to copy, and to represent, requires memory, which is a child's recall of prior knowledge and application of his understanding over time. The time period for application may be short or long term.

Bergen et al. (2018) identified memory potential within every neuron of the brain, and these researchers indicated that emotional development formed a necessary foundation for cognitive skills to accumulate and to refine. Implicit memories are greatly influenced by emotions that accompany an experience, and from birth these memories are stored in the middle and lower part of the brain. Also, during this period of growth is the development of cognition. Enactive cognition entails an infant gaining understanding of the actions of real objects. Iconic cognition entails comprehension of pictures and symbols that represent real objects (Bergen et al., 2018).

Explicit memories are based upon experiential learning and emerge throughout childhood due to dependence on the development of the cerebral cortex (Bergen et al., 2018). Explicit memories may be expressed in the age group of 12 months onwards. By 3 years of age, children have the ability to use their memories voluntarily. Many strategies promote emotional literacy which often entails prompting a young child's memory through discussion, photographs, and actions. Thelen and Smith (2006) conducted research on tasks that used memory. Findings from their study indicated that the ability of a young child to reach and achieve a goal through experiential learning creates a significant long-lasting memory. Experiential play which is supported by an attachment figure is a key response to education in the child's earliest years, and it nurtures conditions for attainment.

Additional learning needs

In a context of children with Down's Syndrome, Fidler (2006) recommended that practitioners promote a child's developmental strengths in order to support weaker areas. Down's Syndrome is a common genetically based syndrome that occurs in approximately one per 700–1,000 births (Bergen et al., 2018). The syndrome is characterised by the existence of an extra chromosome, termed trisomy 21, and it is exhibited by additional support for learning needs. Areas of strength commonly relate to social functioning and the creation of positive relationships, and weaknesses relate to visual processing and visual motor coordination.

Fidler (2006) explains that children with Down's Syndrome have reduced motivation in tasks that are cognitively challenging and demonstrate reliance on social interactions. Fidler described the reduction in motivation to complete tasks as a secondary phenotype that resulted from enhanced primary strengths in social functioning and deficits in instrumental thinking. Instrumental in this context referred to tasks with identified goals. During the first twelve months of childhood, the infants in this study demonstrated a decline in contingency learning compared to the norm.

The use of imaginative skills, often based upon prior knowledge and creativity, can provide potential solutions to challenges during play. Fidler (2006) indicates that infants and preschool children with Down's Syndrome may have difficulty with problem-solving due to a reduced creative ability in comparison to the norm. The research describes how a child with Down's Syndrome accesses his strengths in social interaction by diverting attention from a challenging situation or by recruiting a peer to complete a task.

Evidence from a study by Ruskin et al. (1994) indicates that a young child with Down's Syndrome has difficulties in linking sequences of goal-directed behaviours. Many daily tasks in early years settings involve regular repeated steps which may be implemented on several occasions each session. An example is hand-washing, which has increased in frequency in services as a response to the COVID-19 pandemic. Timelines and photographic prompts are effective, common strategies in supporting every child to recognise, apply, and recall behaviour sequences in order to complete a task.

In busy early years settings, it is not feasible to display personalised prompts for every child, but it is effective practice to use photographs of the child who requires the greatest level of support. Parents can also be encouraged and supported to print out photographic prompts for home use. It is easy to share strategies with families, but it is equally important to determine if families have the means to action these approaches. Additionally, a wall of mirrors situated in front of a child during play or routine tasks can have a major impact upon each child's comprehension of his sense of self. Use of a mirror reinforces the link between cognitive thinking, actions, and behaviour. Viewing one's own image as tasks are completed is an effective approach to support the retention of learning and development of a sense of self.

Ruskin et al. (1994) showed that infants with Down's Syndrome displayed lower levels of causality pleasure than the norm. For example, fewer positive facial displays were observed during tasks that involved the infants using instrumental thinking to problem-solve. Lowered persistence for completing tasks is associated with temperaments that include stubbornness and strong will. The use of targeted and time-sensitive interventions in response to decreased motivation should consider each child's capacity and interest in engaging with specific instrumental tasks. Interests can be used to capture a child's curiosity to explore and to learn, and early years practitioners are skilled in scaffolding and extending development within any context. Fidler (2006) recommended that intervention should be implemented in the earliest days of childhood in order to promote an infant's adaptation to circumstances and to contribute to attainment and independence throughout the lifespan.

Roedell (1984, 1989) commented on significant uneven development in young children who had higher than average ability and emphasised blending of opportunities for social, physical, and emotional development. This researcher also promoted the use of experimentation with manipulative materials as a means to increase visual-motor skills. These media are popular in the early years field for all children. Playdough, gloop, paint, food mixes, and mud kitchens are common features. The rationale for the use of these experiential play activities is broad-ranging, and implementation supports cooperation, social interactions, sensory exploration, imaginative play, hand–eye coordination, gross and fine motor control, and includes the therapeutic value of play in an outdoor green environment.

Tourette's Syndrome is a neuro-developmental disorder which is associated with stereotypical movements and vocalisations. This syndrome tends to become apparent in the middle childhood years, and behavioural symptoms are difficult for the child to control. Bergen et al. (2018) highlight a particular trait linked to children with Tourette's Syndrome as an increased ability to process time. These authors reiterated the message of Fidler (2006) and emphasised the importance of practitioners and parents focusing upon a child's strengths.

Physiological changes have been detected in children who suffer adverse childhood experiences. Patterns of electrical activity in the frontal and temporal lobes are different to the norm. These differences may be exhibited as impulsivity hyperactivity and poor affect regulation as described in the research by Bergen et al. (2018). A previous study, by Bremner et al. (1997), indicated atrophy in the hippocampus of abused children which included long-term memory deficits. These children may react to minor incidents of stress with extreme behaviour, and this can be observed in a nursery setting during play. It is often situations in which the child feels that he has lost control, for example, a social activity requiring cooperative play.

Bergen et al. (2018) studied neural development in children who suffered from the brain condition known as attention-deficit/hyperactivity disorder (ADHD). These authors identified that white and grey matter areas are affected in children who have been diagnosed with this condition, and evidence indicates executive dysfunction and immaturity in frontal-lobe development. The frontal lobe is responsible for regulating and inhibiting actions and planning complex tasks. Panksepp (1998) had closely observed groups of children who had an ADHD diagnosis and noted that their behaviour during play regularly encompassed physical, unplanned movements. Panksepp suggested that extended opportunities for rough-and-tumble play could support frontal-lobe development in children with ADHD. This researcher speculated that drug treatment which induced passivity in children with ADHD could potentially inhibit frontal-lobe development.

Child-led pedagogy

It is so interesting that Panksepp (1998) assumed that children's natural inclination for a particular type of play was a response to their developmental needs. Early years practitioners are trained to observe children during free play, to assess developmental levels and each child's preponderance to particular activities in comparison to the norm. Results are recorded on care plans in the categories of personality, interests, and schemas. Daily observations of children can reveal deficits in development and indicate the body's inherent response to these needs. Interpretation of this information provides a valid baseline for personalised intervention.

Current implementation of curricula is presented within a child-led pedagogy, and children's interests lead the planning and implementation of a learning environment. Greater understanding of these issues can be gained through the research by Panksepp (1998) and the growing awareness in practice of the human body's inherent responses to need by young children's choices of play activities and behaviour. Behaviour may not adhere to social boundaries and expectations of a setting. It is important to provide the child with alternative behavioural choices which continue to respond to needs, including the impact of trauma and social circumstances.

Many years after Panksepp (1998) published his findings, early years settings in many countries provide daily periods of outdoor active play and learning for all children. The therapeutic benefit upon mental health from play within green spaces is recognised by educators and parents. Early years settings provide multiple opportunities for children to develop and to practise skills in a range of environments. Stress can be reduced over time with a therapeutic and nurturing approach which is based upon a secure attachment relationship.

Emotional development and support

Emotions are regarded as responses to external stimuli or internal mental representations based upon the inner working model of an individual. Ochsner and Gross (2005) described emotions as incurring changes within experiential, behavioural, peripheral, and physiological systems. These authors distinguished emotions from moods by relating a trigger to the onset of an emotion. Emotions can be based upon an instinctive response to direct stimuli, or a learned response which may be influenced by prior experiences.

Research studies have shown that infants and young children who have experienced long-term adversity in the form of toxic stress have difficulty in identifying emotions through facial expressions. It is also suggested that emotional discrimination ability is affected by the type of abuse which the child has suffered. Pollak et al. (2000) indicated that neglected children had the greatest difficulty in discriminating between facial expressions compared to children who had experienced physical abuse. The latter group of children demonstrated a noticeable response to angry expressions compared to other negative emotions.

Research indicates three significant aspects which have emerged through studies of emotion regulation and cognitive control. Ochsner and Gross (2005) describe these aspects as:

1   Defence mechanisms.
2   Management of situations that exceed the resources of an individual.
3   Self-regulation in a context of socio-emotional development.

This study investigated the impact of behavioural or cognitive regulation (Ochsner & Gross, 2005). A significant finding indicated that regulation of behaviour associated with negative emotions would limit the individual's actions. However, the regulation did not reduce the negative emotional experiences which were retained as memories after an event. For example, children can learn to adhere to social boundaries while continuing to experience an emotional impact which is triggered by memory of negative influences.

Alternatively, cognitive regulation can reduce the negative emotional impact and, potentially, the physiological effects. Cognitive regulation is sectioned into two strands: attentional control and cognitive change. The study by Ochsner and Gross (2005) revealed marked variability in the type and impact of emotional responses from participants. Links were indicated between gender, personality, negative affectivity, and regulatory ability.

Structural and functional changes in control and appraisal systems in children may influence emotional responses. Additionally, abilities are dependent upon interactions between prefrontal systems that support control processes and posterior cortical and subcortical systems that represent different types of modality, for example, visual, spatial, and auditory information (Ochsner & Gross, 2005). Modulation of appraisal systems can be influenced by first supporting an infant or child to reinterpret stimuli and promote meaning that engenders different emotions; and, second, to associate a different emotional response to the same stimuli. Attachment figures in services and the home environment can provide effective role models in supporting a child to reconfigure previous understanding of stimuli and emotions.

Many opportunities occur within daily living to promote emotional literacy and to contribute to positive infant mental health. Therapeutic approaches are regularly used within early years settings to support emotional needs and include activation of the child's higher cognitive abilities, for example, promoting the use of working memory, long-term memory, and mental recall. These abilities support reappraisal of one's own emotional reactions, and behaviour.

Specific interventions of play therapy have been commonly implemented within services in response to mental-health issues, particularly in the past two decades. It is inciteful to gain understanding from the study by Ritzi and Ray (2017) on play therapy. These authors associated reflection on emotional events with an enhanced ability to increase or to decrease amygdala responses. The intervention of play therapy enabled the children to reappraise their emotional responses and to alter their behaviour accordingly.

Neural changes and abuse

Childhood abuse has a long-term impact upon mental health and overall development. During this period, the brain's development encompasses synaptic remodelling, myelination, and cell death which affects the organisation of the grey and the white matter. Hart and Rubia (2012) indicated that adverse childhood experiences could result in physiological, neurochemical, and hormonal changes that altered brain structure and, ultimately, neural functioning. These authors described modulation changes by the serotonin system, sympathetic nervous system, and the hypothalamic-pituitary adrenal axis. Findings indicated internal behavioural problems as reduced tolerance for stress, anxiety, affective instability, depression, suicidality, and post-traumatic stress disorder. External behavioural symptoms include limited impulse control, episodic aggression, substance abuse, ADHD, and conduct disorder.

Ochsner and Gross (2005) linked disruption in the development of the fronto-limbic neural circuits to effects from childhood that can endure throughout adulthood. For example, motor control, memory, emotion regulation, and ability to learn social behaviours. However, the findings of Hart and Rubia (2012) showed that emotion discrimination can improve through time. A child's understanding of his own emotions, and others, is a key element of the curriculum in an early years service and promotion of broad experiences contribute to maturation in childhood, and beyond.

Studies have found that the volume of the brain is affected by a child's age at the onset of trauma and duration of abuse (Hart & Rubia, 2012). Neuroimaging of the brains of children who had been known to suffer abuse demonstrated brain structural differences compared to the norm. The imaging was associated with limitations in memory, working memory, attention, response inhibition, and emotion discrimination. The neuroimages showed reduction in the brain volume and the grey and white matter distribution in the dorsolateral and ventromedial prefrontal cortex, hippocampus, amygdala, and corpus callosum. In addition, diffusion tensor imaging revealed deficiencies in the neural networks. Research can give great insight into children's mental health, an acute awareness of the impact of various levels of stress upon each child, and increase understanding of actions, reactions, and intervention routes.

McCrory et al. (2011) also identified differences in the corpus callosum of children who had experienced abuse and variations in the hippocampus of adults who had experienced adversities in childhood. The study described amygdala hyperactivity and atypical activation of frontal regions in the adults. The findings indicated a direct link between abuse, brain structure, and the impact from gene–environment interaction. It was reported that specific genotypes may moderate the association between childhood maltreatment and psychopathology.

Research by Bergen et al. (2018) revealed different patterns of electrical activity in the temporal and frontal lobes of abused children in comparison to the norm. It is known that abused children can exhibit extraordinary physiological responses to minor issues. Research indicates that trauma affects the brainstem areas that regulate these physiological responses relating to survival (Perry, 1997). Alongside this overdevelopment of the brainstem areas, Perry identified restriction in development of the corticol and the limbic areas that control higher-order thinking and emotions. Bremner et al. (2008) also investigated these topics, and findings showed that the hippocampus may be atrophied in children who have experienced abuse. This defect can impact upon long-term memory; however, an enriched environment can promote hippocampal neurogenesis.

Perry (1997) describes the human brain as an organ that processes information from inside and outside the body in order to act and to ensure survival. The lower areas of the brain encapsulate the brainstem and midbrain which maintain simple regulatory functions, for example, heart rate, body temperature, and blood pressure. It is within higher areas of the brain that complex functions are maintained, for example, the use of language and abstract cognition. This hierarchy of activity begins pre-birth, and the main structural organisation is formed throughout childhood.

It is enlightening to read Perry's explanation of the neurobiology of violence. Perry (1997) explored neurodevelopment, violence, and potential influences, and this author determined that experience has the greatest impact upon human behaviour. Perry clearly states that genetics do not result in the neurobiological factors which are commonly associated with violence. Findings from this study indicated that violence, aggression, and impulsivity are closely linked to an increase in reactivity of the brainstem as a result of toxic stress and a decrease in the moderation capacity of the limbic or cortical areas. This decrease can be influenced by adversities associated with neglect.

The study described the brain's impulse-mediating capacity as relating to activity in the lower primitive parts of the brain *and* activity in the higher cortical areas.

It is well documented that there are critical and sensitive periods for development in which the brain gains optimum value from learning experiences with a focus upon sensory input (Perry, 1997). Any atypical patterns of neural activity during these periods can impact negatively upon functions throughout the lifespan such as empathy, affect regulation, and attachment. Perry linked emotional neglect in childhood to violence in adulthood by identifying a decrease in strength of the subcortical and cortical impulse-modulation capacities. The research also highlighted a limited ability to empathise or sympathise with others. Perry associates the use of alcohol or drugs with negative attitude and physical violence in late childhood and adulthood. This author explained that intoxicating agents can further reduce the ability to control oneself physically and emotionally and for individuals who already have reduced capacity then the outcome may incur aggression and violence.

The aforementioned explanation of neural workings is complex and challenging to relate to practice knowledge in order to enhance the day-to-day delivery of a service. However, Perry (1997) highlights moderating capacity as a key neurodevelopmental factor that provides a target area for intervention. Each child's capacity to moderate his actions and reactions can be increased by an adult supporting consolidation and change in the child's inner working model. Exposure to curricular and home experiences and a secure attachment relationship are key contributions to the change process in this context.

Time-dependent and experience-dependent

Organisation of the neural networks is time-dependent or experience-dependent. Any disruptions can result in abnormalities or deficits in neurodevelopment. Perry (1997) relates disruptions to a lack of sensory experiences during critical periods of development, or the direct impact of adversities upon the infant. The research emphasises the sequential development of the brain as a critical factor in the impact of disruptions. Findings indicated that adversities in early childhood, including the perinatal period, can alter development of the brainstem or midbrain and subsequently impact upon the limbic and cortical development.

It is useful to visualise this hierarchy of developmental stages as building upon a solid foundational base of knowledge and understanding which is provided by learning opportunities in the early years. Practitioners are taught to assess and to respond to a child's stage of development as opposed to using age-appropriate activities. This approach to early learning and development is an essential factor in supporting the incremental stages of neural development, and practice should focus upon relationships, opportunities, and environment.

Quality and breadth of experiences have direct relevance to growth of the human cortex; therefore, a lack of sensory-motor and cognitive opportunities reduces potential for development. The research of Perry (1997) highlighted smaller cortical and subcortical areas linked to neglect of children. The term "cortical atrophy", as used by Perry, referred to underuse of the cortical areas and subsequently underdevelopment. Infants who exist in adversity present as hypervigilant and unusually sensitive to external stimuli. Perry indicated that this group of infants and children tend to focus upon non-verbal communication cues, in a context of survival. Limitations on cognitive thinking can reduce cortical growth. Findings revealed an increase in muscle tone, a greater startle response, unusual sleep patterns, affect regulation issues, anxiety, and abnormal cardiovascular regulation in the participant group.

Aggressive behaviour gives the child perceived or actual control over his environment, which is an inherent reaction to threat. The child is seeking a predictable response from another person in order to prevent or to control potentially harmful interactions. Early years services promote nurturing caring learning contexts, but the neglected infant may interpret tentative overtures from peers or practitioners as a prelude to abuse. Repeated observation and interpretation of the child's emotional, behavioural, cognitive, social, and physiological functioning, in the broad influential context of home, service, and the community, are necessary responses. Practitioners should apply this information to support sensitive responding through an attachment relationship and appropriate environmental stimulus. Engaging with a stressed child and supporting containment of his aggression is the first step of a therapeutic approach. Over time, the child gains patterns of skills that allow him to refocus his reaction to non-verbal indicators, to verbal reflection, cognitive solutions, and ultimately reconfiguration of the inner working model.

Green spaces

Early years services use sensory activities as a medium for promoting the development of children from birth to three years of age (Scottish Government, 2010). An increase in comprehension of the rationale of this approach can transform the impetus, motivation, and creativity of practitioners in teaching and caring for our youngest learners. Once again, research findings highlight the importance of curriculum planning and implementation of a rich learning environment that nurtures optimum capacity of the neural areas of each child.

Robinson and Brown (2016) referred to the use of outdoor spaces to induce a calm, ambient atmosphere. Green exercise was the term applied by Barton and Pretty (2010) within research using data from adult participants. The study compared short- and long-term health benefits that could be gained from an outdoor environment. Findings indicated that the greatest positive changes were demonstrated by the youngest participants who had existing mental-health conditions.

Louv (2005) applied the descriptor "nature-deficit disorder" to indicate the negative effects that relate to lack of outdoor stimulation in the context of urban dwellings. Jawer (2005) reviewed the topic from the young child's perspective, and he suggested that environmental sensitivity can be nurtured through the provision of outdoor play opportunities. Outcomes for the child represent outcomes for nature. The child's understanding of himself as relevant, respected, and looked after by society, is gained through his comprehension and response to the natural world (Whitters, 2019).

Ohly et al. (2016) explain this phenomenon in the context of attention restoration theory. A literature review of 31 studies had been used to investigate attention fatigue, which is a condition associated with low self-regulation, poor decision-making, and physical ill-health. Findings indicated that ability and capacity to concentrate and to increase executive functioning can be restored through exposure to natural environments.

Attention restoration theory explains the ability and capacity to refocus and increase attention to learning in four categories (Kaplan, 1995):

1   Short-term respite from daily adversities.
2   Exposure to broader contexts of living through interactions within enhanced spaces.
3   Opportunities to follow personal interests and respond to needs.
4   Experiencing stimuli that do not impose demands upon the individual.

The principles of fascination, compatibility, and extension traverse the four categories as described by Kaplan (1995). Kaplan made an important distinction between hard fascination and soft fascination. Hard fascination activities tend to have identifiable goals and one outcome for the participant is an increase in stimulation of the human senses that may incur a physiological reaction such as rapid heartbeat and a feeling of dejection or euphoria. Soft fascination activities may not have a specific goal. The outcome for the participant occurs within a period of reflection which includes a restorative effect upon the human body, an increase in awareness of self and potentially appreciation of the wonder of nature.

Box 5.1 Example from practice

Attention restoration theory in practice: two young friends are supported to don green rubber boots and striped blue and red waterproof jackets for garden play in their local nursery garden. Glory and Lewis are 2½ years old, a significant age of development in which the infant has progressed through the toddler stage and is entering a period in which competence and a sense of self increase markedly. The garden is also experiencing an important transformation in this penultimate season of the year. Autumn is a time of endings and beginnings. Orange, brown, and green leaves tumble down in unpredictable spirals to land softly upon the sodden withered grass. Rubber matting surrounds the apple tree swing to maintain a semblance of dry ground for intrepid adventurers. Miniature green shoots can already be spotted peeping around the edges of the rubber mats, responding to a few days of mild weather. Papers and sundry refuse items have escaped from the large industrial metal bins, and the wind encourages these items to fly across and over the garden, high into the dark sky, and beyond the rooftops.

Glory and Lewis are best friends. They share a passion for energetic play, for digging in a mud kitchen, for exploring familiar corners of the garden, and hiding excitedly in the long bamboo grasses. Lewis always has a goal, and he uses this green space to further his interests. Currently his play focuses upon building upwards, and along. The garden offers ample materials for this constructor of ideas, and he works industriously and individually by gathering wooden bricks and freeze blocks. The child stands back to survey his preparations, and he puts a plan into action. It looks like this little boy is constructing a tower. Lewis could be described as experiencing hard fascination within the outdoor environment. He builds upwards and along the winding path which is strewn with bark pieces. His plan changes and adapts to the materials and to his ability in creating a stable structure. As the thin tower cascades to the ground, Lewis giggles, his plan has changed instantaneously, and his new goal has been achieved.

Glory is sitting under a bush. The rhododendron creates a tent-like canopy of dark green foliage above the little girl's head, and isolated drips of rain disrupt her play flow, just momentarily. Glory has a worm in the palm of her hand. The long slender worm is unsure of this new warm environment. He lifts his head and waves it around to detect familiar territory. Glory touches the worm with a fingertip, and he retracts quickly, curling tightly upon her palm. The movements feel like gentle tickling to this young explorer. The child waits and watches – a silent learner. Glory is experiencing soft fascination within her nurturing bush corner in the nursery garden.

A later study by Kaplan and Berman (2010) identified two types of attention: voluntary and involuntary. Voluntary attention is currently termed "directed attention", and it relates to a child's conscious focus upon an activity. Involuntary attention requires less concerted effort due to a specific interest of the child being met or attraction to the content through curiosity or prior knowledge. An outdoor environment is commonly regarded as a context in which children and adults demonstrate involuntary attention; however, the restoration effect from interaction within green spaces can also support directed attention associated with specific plans and goals.

Good health and attainment were linked by Kuo and Taylor (2004) within a study upon play within green spaces. Findings indicated that symptoms associated with attention fatigue, which is a periodic condition, were similar to characteristics of ADHD, which is a long-term condition. Conclusions reported that direct interaction within green spaces, or indirect pictorial representations linked to attainment in activities which immediately followed these experiences. Findings concluded that exercise in green spaces reduced the characteristics of attention fatigue and increased the capacity for learning that occurred after the physical activity. Many settings incorporate physical play outdoors during the initial period of a session. Anecdotal comments by parents declare that "Children learn better if they run off their energy first!" Outdoor play stimulates the physical body, and mind, in addition to enveloping a child in the therapeutic atmosphere of a natural space.

The data of 175 participants, which was collated in a study by Corraliza et al. (2012), had indicated that children who were exposed to nature on a regular basis had increased coping strategies in response to adversities. Interestingly, in this study, the children who were most vulnerable experienced the greatest positive effects from contact with the natural environment.

Since I have been studying research, I have realised that findings can often be given clarity by linking to practical experiences in the field. Research informs practice by presenting rationale, knowledge based upon theory, and findings gained within a formal context of information retrieval. Practical experience educates the practitioner by presenting understanding and application of knowledge in situ. Research and practice should be regarded as interdependent and equally valuable for professional development.

It is important for early years practitioners to liaise with parents in order to analyse characteristics that aid attention restoration and to reflect the cultural context of the area, for example, urban or rural, and needs of service-users. Strategies can be actioned through effective professional–parent partnerships and consistent communication links between service and home environment. Facebook pages are currently popular media for sharing ideas between service-providers and service-users. An increase in the use of social media has led to many services using instructional videos to encourage and to support parent–child interaction within a family home. Videos present a role model for parents and children to copy. It may be that the parent provides a learning medium by copying the interactions from the video, and the child copies his parent. Alternatively, child and parent may jointly use the video as their source of role-modelling.

Capacity

Capacity relates to emotional well-being, which is founded on a child's secure attachment with one or more adults, and it increases alongside a child's resilience to adversities. The current term which is being used in childcare is "homeostasis" (National Scientific Council on the Developing Child, 2020). This descriptor is representative of a child having optimal emotional well-being and resilience that leads to demonstration of motivation and curiosity to seek out learning opportunities. Stern (1998) describes daily social interactions and care routines as major contributions to this status of a young child.

Increasing capacity includes an infant learning by gaining knowledge and understanding of the world through the medium of his senses: sight, hearing, smell, taste, and touch. Emotional well-being is a necessary condition for a child to liberate his five senses for learning that leads to development. If a child is suffering from internal stresses, then he may appear vigilant and alert for danger to himself, even within the safe environment of a nursery. The receptivity of his five senses becomes heightened. Being alert is a basic survival instinct, and, although a child's senses are attuned and primed to gain understanding of the proximal environment, it is for the purpose of detecting danger as opposed to development.

Bowlby (1997) recorded different forms of behaviour that linked to attachment status:

- Interactive behaviour with mother, which includes physical contact.
- Responses to mother's interactions.
- Behaviour that attempts to avoid separation from mother.
- Behaviour on reunion with mother which includes greeting responses, avoidance, rejection, or ambivalence.
- Withdrawal behaviour based upon fear.
- Exploratory behaviour which is orientated towards the mother.

Bowlby (1997) described exploratory behaviour by focusing upon three actions. The infant moves his head and body into a position that prepares muscles and cardiovascular system for action, the senses are primed to seek out and to process information, and, finally, manipulation of an object commences which is led by curiosity. This behavioural system is led or stopped by stimuli with particular characteristics relating to novelty and familiarity. Exploration and learning transform a novel object into a familiar one.

Play cycle

King and Sturrock (2020) identified four levels of intervention which could be implemented to support a play cycle:

- Play maintenance in which the adult observes the activity. I would add that the adult presents a positive attitude and demonstrates an interested focus upon the child's play.
- Simple intervention in which the adult can suggest uses for the resources. The key term indicates the adult should not lead the play cycle.
- Medial intervention in which the adult is invited to participate by the child. I add that the adult suggests ideas for the play but takes direction from the child and responds promptly to his play cues, and to his emotional reactions.
- Complex intervention in which the adult becomes intertwined in the child's play cycle. Reciprocal interactions can occur in this context, but the adult should continue to overtly recognise the child as the director of his play.

Freeman (1998) indicated that negative emotions can inhibit curiosity in accordance with findings from an extensive German study on children. Divergent thinking will not occur if a child's capacity is lowered. Adversities may have a short-term effect upon capacity to learn, or detrimentally affect a child's lifestyle on a long-term basis. Interruption of a play cycle was described by King and Temple (2020) as resulting in dysplay and this hiatus in learning was linked directly to negative emotional reactions. During observations in a playroom practitioners should consider whether the play cycle is interrupted by an internal emotional influence from within the infant which is based upon memory, or an external factor that leads to this emotional barrier. An infant who is reacting to an external source will usually turn towards that source, for example, a loud noise in the vicinity, or deliberately turn away from a local source, for example, another child screaming.

In early years settings and the home environment, children may demonstrate emotional reactions when their play cycle is curtailed, for example, crying, shouting, aggressive behaviour, or quiet emotional withdrawal. The child's homeostasis becomes uneven. There are many valid reasons for shortening a play cycle, particularly within a service that is encompassed by the necessity of routines. However, the key to responsive support by an adult is preparing the child for ending a play cycle and by introducing transitional strategies that lead towards the next event. Preparation is a valuable approach that facilitates a child's emotional and physical adaptation to situations. I observe young children in nurseries completing their play cycle rapidly after being informed that "tidy-up time" will commence in a few minutes. Practitioners can support the ending of a play cycle through verbal tracking of the child's actions and encouragement to look forward to the next activity or event.

One important component of learning is delivery of knowledge in a manner and medium that promotes understanding by each recipient. Instruction needs to be on par with the developmental level of the individual child and to be accompanied by motivational prompts that match his personality, needs, and interests at a point in time. The research of McCoach and Flake (2018) indicated that frequent praise in relation to achievement may impact negatively upon a child's resilience. Zhou and Brown (2015) had referred to a self-ranking system in which a child may gain a sense of the autobiographical self as good or bad; thus, the child's sense of self is inadvertently linked to adult or peer feedback. Motivation is reliant on an external source. Harter (2006) commented that abuse in childhood can result in the child viewing himself as bad, and this writer linked adverse circumstances to depression in the early years.

Ability may not be demonstrated consistently by a child due to internal and external influences upon the learner. Hypervigilance can direct a baby or young child's attention away from his learning needs, and interests. Mental health, personality, and environment, which is conducive to the child's interests, are factors that can strongly impact upon application and, consequently, demonstration of ability.

Task commitment is represented by motivation to focus upon a specific problem or area in which understanding is being sought (Renzulli & Reis, 2018). Descriptors which are used in association with this cluster are "dedication", "endurance", and "self-confidence". Task commitment is underpinned by the child's sense of self, albeit at a rudimentary stage in earliest childhood, which includes being a physical, social, and teleological agent (Whitters, 2019).

Harter (2006) presents a parental responsibility as supporting a child to develop a narrative of self, for example, a positive representation of childhood as recorded in photographs, memory stories of significant events, and cultural routines pertaining to each family. This narrative includes perceptions and interpretation of the world from a young child's viewpoint in addition to parental interpretation or other dominant adults. Harter used the term "impoverished self" to represent the outcome of a parent's failure to support the child's creation of a positive narrative of self. Application that demonstrates commitment by a parent will support a child to understand his fourth level of self as an intentional mental agent. An elementary level of the autobiographical self is generally achieved within the first five years; however, environmental and social adversities may hinder this stage of development.

During parenting work, I find that many parents and children who live in adversity require sensitive prompting and probing questions in order to recall positive memories of the early days of their lives. Creating a narrative of self is a significant stage of childhood that affects early and middle childhood, adolescence, adulthood, and parental identity. Interventions must support this foundational aspect of development. Harter (2006) emphasised the importance of creating an autobiographical memory which influences hopes and dreams for the future. Creativity is linked to the sense of self, and this trait is only fully liberated when an autobiographical self is understood and embraced by the individual.

Creativity

Creativity involves devising and following a plan that leads to a unique outcome. There are numerous skill sets associated with planning and implementation of self-appointed goals by children. Plucker and Barab (2005) describe creativity as interaction between environment, process, and a child's aptitude, and, finally the acknowledgement of an end goal. These authors did comment that creativity may be directed by cultural influences and led by expectations of adults, in addition to the child's own goals.

Creativity requires imagination and an ability and desire to extrapolate beyond the status quo. A point of clarification is made by Renzulli (2019) as he does not exclusively link creativity to process and production of an end goal. This author includes descriptors of creativity as originality of thought, receptivity to new experiences, curiosity within a learning environment, sensitivity to detail, and awareness of the emotions of self and others. In the early years services, these descriptors are commonly used to understand and to assess children's progress in a context of curriculum delivery and to guide practitioners in planning a rich learning environment.

It is interesting that Kayal (2020) mentions links between creativity and the child's relationships with teachers and parents. The impact from relationships upon learning indicates that development can be supported within formal and informal environments which may have different cultures. Culture can exist within a local setting, such as a family home or nursery, or it can be associated with a particular talent or embedded within the expectations of a nation. Creativity should be embraced and used to forge links between areas of learning. Diversity among siblings and peers should be celebrated in order to recognise unique attributes as positive.

Csikszentmihalyi et al. (2018) emphasised the complexity of the psychological aspects of flow theory and applied the systems model of creativity to promote understanding. A cyclical process occurs as a child experiences flow theory. He uses intrinsic motivation to achieve goals which are based upon creative ideas. This theory indicates that genes may predispose an individual to a high level of learning, but creativity is regarded as a social construction that embraces all stages of cognitive development. Creativity is recognised as a child learning and demonstrating application of existing domain knowledge which is enriched by his original ideas. Prior knowledge in a particular domain provides a framework for the scaffolding of creativity. Csikszentmihalyi et al. (2018) commented that creativity may be identified within a specific context through demonstration of cultural relevance and improvement to a child's previous creations.

Opportunities for creativity are regularly incorporated within parenting programmes and also support primary carers to explore their own identity which is based upon interests, needs, and spontaneous ideas. The National Scientific Council on the Developing Child (2020) recently published research that portrays the importance of brain development in the pre-natal period and postnatal years of life to long-term success and health in adulthood. The conclusion of this investigation declares that it is never too late to reduce risk to development. This research upholds the implementation of parenting work by services with members of the extended family, for example, a third generation in the context of grandparents.

Individuality and developmental progress can be observed by the adaptations of children and adults to situations and evidence of their maturity and experience during ongoing interactions with the environment. An opposing influence upon developmental progress is resistance to change (Rathunde & Csikszentmihalyi, 2006). Rathunde and Csikszentmihalyi described equilibrium in human systems as being affected by boredom and anxiety. An individual can overcome boredom by seeking out challenges, and he can overcome anxiety by increasing skills and resilience which give him greater choices and a sense of control. The former entails creativity within a process of seeking novelty. The latter entails problem-solving and reliance upon current skills or scaffolding which culminates in an increase in understanding.

The following two studies illustrate the importance of the adult–child relationship to a young child's interpretation, understanding, and involvement within a learning environment (Bernier et al., 2012; Nermeen et al., 2010). In 2012, Bernier and a research team identified three distinct dimensions of parental involvement with their children's learning in the formative years:

1   Sensitive responding.
2   Mindfulness.
3   Promotion of the child's autonomy.

The study focused upon children from birth to 2 years. The brain grows rapidly during the first two years of life, and it attains 90 per cent of the size of an adult brain during this period. The findings indicated that stimulation during the first two years directly impacted the infant's frontal brain development. Additionally, mindfulness of a parent enhanced the response to an infant and supported his self-regulation within contexts of emotionally challenging situations. The research concluded that infants, who are securely attached to a primary carer, are more competent in transferring their skill sets to circumstances out-with the dyadic relationship.

Nermeen et al. (2010) conducted research on potential links between parental involvement and academic and social development in the early stage of school attendance. Findings indicated that if parents adopted the values and expectations of a school then there was a direct and positive impact upon their child's behaviour. Consistency and continuity of expectations and boundaries were also key influences that supported children's autonomy. The authors suggested that an indirect impact may result from an increase in the child's motivation to engage with learning and a subsequent increase in academic achievement.

Acceleration and enrichment

Two approaches were used to promote development of children 30 years ago in the form of acceleration or enrichment. The rationale of using acceleration or enrichment is to promote three levels of thinking: divergent, convergent, and evaluative. In early years services, play spaces are bound by adult to child ratios and formal registration of each area in accordance with a specific age group. Acceleration of learning, by moving a child from chronological age group to a playroom with older peers, may not be achievable within registration policies. Additionally, greater comprehension has been gained over the past 30 years of the significance of emotional development in a context of learning and attainment. The passing of time, a secure attachment to an adult, and exposure to a range of experiences, are factors that directly affect maturation of a child's emotional literacy. A child with a higher than average level of ability may embrace the cognitive stimulation and challenges which are presented within an older age group; however, his level of emotional development may not be sufficient to cope with the complexity of social interactions. Currently, enrichment tends to be the more common approach to promoting children's development.

Divergent thinking

Divergent thinking leads to a new base of knowledge and understanding from an original foundation termed the child's inner working model, as described by Bowlby (1997). As a child explores an environment, or a concept, he uses information from his current inner working model to interpret, and to respond. The child's memory, and imagination, are activated during these processes, and neural links are made to prior knowledge on similar topics. Cognitive skill supports the brain to merge these links, and to formulate new ideas that lead to the child interpreting the concept from a different perspective. This new perspective reconfigures the child's inner working model, and his original foundation of knowledge and understanding alters. Rathunde & Csikszentmihalyi (2006) used the term "creative thinking" to describe the various steps and "closure" to indicate completion of this cognitive process. In an early years setting, it is important that children are offered multiple choices of materials to support divergent thinking, and creativity. Choices should always include familiar and unfamiliar items.

Box 5.2 Example from practice

Natalia and Mehwish started nursery on the same day. These two 4-year-old girls have been placed together in the Yellow Group and share a key worker. It is fascinating to observe friendships emerging in young children. This is an area of development which is the child's own domain. Key workers may offer opportunities of partnership activities or set out furniture and toys to encourage cooperative play and turn-taking of resources; however, the creation of a peer relationship is incited by a child's personality and nurtured by her emotional well-being.

Mehwish enters the playroom and scans the corners for her friend. The room is quiet at this point. Families follow timetables based upon lifestyles, and every practitioner is well aware of the early birds in nursery and the latecomers who have to be gently integrated into breakfast routines which are already ongoing in the nursery. Natalia and Mehwish are always early, and ready to learn. Both children chose to bypass the breakfast choices and marched determinedly towards an unfamiliar box. The tall cardboard box is sitting squarely in the middle of the jungle corner. Yesterday, this box was the receptacle for nursery supplies. Today, it promises to expose a myriad of exciting artefacts in the playroom. Recycling not only helps the environment but also provides stimulating challenges for developing youngsters.

The jungle is an area which has been transformed by a creative early years student: multiple green and yellow paper strands curl downwards and across the corner to create a hideout. Large soft rubber animals nestle in amongst a mat of artificial wiry grass: elephants, tigers, giraffes, hippopotamus, crocodiles, and a solitary sheep which has escaped from the farm box. The surface has been dotted with round ladybird leaves that act as little seats for the children.

The two friends peep into the box and open their eyes wide as they exchange excited glances. Mehwish jumps up and down, and the intrepid Natalia stretches her hand to retrieve some kitchen-roll holders. In seconds, she has placed a holder onto the head of each animal, obscuring their faces, and Natalia declares to her peer, "Putting on their hats." There is no need for the girls in this learning partnership to use long sentences as the core information is shared. Additionally, communication between friends always contains understanding which is sourced from knowledge of one another and the focus upon shared interests. Mehwish nods vigorously in agreement, and the little girl covers her eyes as she laughs, "They can't see any more." Divergent thinking in an instance.

Convergent thinking

Convergent thinking occurs when the brain identifies similarities in knowledge and understanding of an environment or concept in relation to previous experience. This array of information from the child's inner working model is sorted and merged during problem-solving to result in a consensus. A young child can be observed in a nursery, or home setting using this base of information to influence his response to a practical problem. Key workers or parents can often recall past experiences which have informed a child's inner working model and subsequently lead to a demonstration of convergent thinking. In an early years setting, this understanding of a child's learning processes is important to inform curricular planning and implementation within a playroom or outdoor setting.

During the past two decades, the presentation of educational choices that respond to children's interests has been identified as a significant influence upon engagement and involvement with learning. Reflection on evidence-gathering and identification of links to progress are essential aspects of professional development. Planning an environment to support delivery of a curriculum, and ultimately attainment, is a key skill within the early years services. Regular records by key workers on each child's progress should be one aspect of evidence-gathering that can be linked directly to a curriculum room planner and evaluation of provision for each child in addition to assessment of the overall service.

Lloyd and Howe (2003) conducted a study on potential links between different types of solitary play and convergent or divergent thinking. There are many factors that can lead a child to choose solitary play: age and stage of development, environmental prompts, personality, adversity, or lower and higher ability than peers. Solitary play was categorised by these authors into three aspects: active, passive, or reticent, in which the child demonstrated little emotion. Participants in this study were 72 children aged 4½ years of age. Findings indicated that active solitary play was positively associated with divergent thinking. Solitary play that was accompanied by reticent behaviour was negatively associated with convergent and divergent thinking. This study indicates that children demonstrate divergent thinking through use of intrinsic motivation, as portrayed by this research context of active solitary play, and creativity.

Evaluative thinking

Evaluative thinking relates to a child taking time away from practical inter-action, albeit momentarily, to reflect upon newly acquired knowledge and understanding. The evaluative process supports creation of memories and retention of information as patterns of exploration and problem-solving. Neural networks need time and appropriate conditions to make connections, and busy, noisy playrooms are not always conducive to evaluative thinking. Breakout areas, for example, tents and quiet corners, and reducing the intru-sion of external noises, can positively influence evaluative thinking in young children. Specific periods for evaluation are incorporated into education and care settings and termed thinking and recall times.

Runco (1991) conducted an interesting study in the 1990s, in which he researched evaluative thinking with over 100 young schoolchildren. This researcher wanted to determine if the use of creativity was intentional or unintentional. It seems that creativity is intentional if shown to link with evaluative thinking by a child. Findings indicated correlation between diver-gent thinking which inherently involved creativity and evaluative ability. Additionally, it was noted that evaluation by a child was influenced positively by a teacher's questions. This finding suggests that open questioning can be used as a positive strategy to promote evaluation as an aspect of learning. Reflection spaces, circle time, news time, and nurture groups are current descriptors of practical responses which are commonly used in early years settings and primary schools. These strategies encourage divergent thinking, creativity, and evaluative ability.

References

Barton, J., & Pretty, J. (2010). What is the best dose of nature and green exercise for improving mental health? A multi-study analysis. *Environmental Science Technol-ogy*, 44(*10*), 3947–3955.

Bergen, D., Schroer, J., & Woodin, M. (2018). *Brain research in education and the social sciences: Implications for practice, parenting, and future society*. Abingdon and New York: Routledge.

Bernier, A., Carlson, S., Deschenes, M., & Matt-Gagne, C. (2012). Social factors in the development of early executive functioning: A closer look at the caregiving environment. *Developmental Science*, 15(*1*), 12–24.

Blumenfeld, P. C., Marx, R., & Harris, C. J. (2006). Learning environments. In W. Damon & R. M. Lerner (Eds.), *Handbook of child psychology*, vol. IV, *Child psychology in practice* (pp. 297–342). Hoboken, NJ: John Wiley & Sons.

Bowlby, J. (1997). *Attachment and loss.* London: Pimlico.

Bremner, J. D., Elzinga, B., Schmahl, C., & Vermetten, E. (2008). Structural and functional plasticity of the human brain in posttraumatic stress disorder. *Progress in Brain Research*, 167, 171–186.

Bremner, J. D., Randall, I. P., Vermetten, E., Staib, L., Bronen, R. A., Mazure, C., Capelli, S., McCarthy, G., Innis, R. B., & Charney, D. S. (1997). Magnetic resonance imaging-based measurement of hippocampal volume in posttraumatic stress disorder related to childhood physical and sexual abuse: A preliminary report. *Biological Psychiatry*, 41(1), 23–32.

Corraliza, J. A., Collado, S., & Bethelmy, L. (2012). Nature as a moderator of stress in urban children. *Social and Behavioural Sciences*, 38, 253–263.

Csikszentmihalyi, M., Montijo, M. N., & Mouton, A. R. (2018). Flow theory: Optimising elite performance in the creative realm. In S. I. Pfeiffer (Ed.), *APA handbook of giftedness and talent* (pp. 215–229). Washington, DC: American Psychological Association.

Fidler, D. (2006). The emergence of a syndrome-specific personality profile in young children with Down syndrome. *Down Syndrome Research and Practice*, 10(2), 53–60.

Fosha, D. (2003). Dyadic regulation and experiential work with emotion and relatedness in trauma and disorganised attachment. In M. F. Solomon & D. J. Siegel (Eds.), *Healing trauma: Attachment, mind, body, and brain.* London: W. W. Norton & Company.

Freeman, J. (1998). *Educating the very able: Current international research.* London: The Stationery Office.

Hart, H., & Rubia, K. (2012). Neuroimaging of child abuse: A critical review. *Frontiers in human neuroscience.* https://www.frontiersin.org/articles/10.3389/fnhum.2012.00052/full.

Harter, S. (2006). The self. In W. Damon & R. M. Lerner (Eds.), *Handbook of child psychology: Social, emotional, and personality development* (pp. 505–570). Hoboken, NJ: Wiley & Sons.

Jawer, M. (2005). Environmental sensitivity: A neurobiological phenomenon? *Seminars in Integrative Medicine* 3(3), 104–109. https://www.researchgate.net/publication/222409869_Environmental_Sensitivity_A_Neurobiological_Phenomenon.

Kaplan, S. (1995). The restorative benefits of nature: Toward an integrative framework. *Journal of Environmental Psychology*, 15, 169–182.

Kaplan, S., & Berman, M. (2010). Executive function and self-regulation. *Association for Psychological Science*, 5(*1*), 43–57.

Kayal, N. G. (2020) Supporting of gifted children's psychosocial developments in preschool period. *Psychology Research on Education and Social Sciences* 1(1), 25–30.

King, P., & Sturrock, G. (2020). *The play cycle: Theory, research, and application.* Abingdon and New York: Routledge.

King, P., & Temple, S. (2020). A review of the play cycle. In P. King & G. Sturrock (Eds.), *The play cycle: theory, research, and application* (pp. 14–38). Abingdon and New York: Routledge.

Kuo, F. E., & Taylor, A. F. (2004). A potential natural treatment for attention-deficit/ hyperactivity disorder: Evidence from a national study. *American Journal of Public Health*, 94 (9), 1580–1586.

Lloyd, B., & Howe, N. (2003). Solitary play and convergent and divergent thinking skills in preschool children. *Early Childhood Research Quarterly*, 18(1), 22–41.

Louv, R. (2005). *Last child in the woods: Saving our children from nature-deficit disorder*. New York: Algonquin Books of Chapel Hill.

McCoach, D. B., & Flake, J. K. (2018). The role of motivation. In S. I. Pfeiffer (Ed.), *APA handbook of giftedness and talent* (pp. 201–213). Washington, DC: American Psychological Association.

McCrory, E., De Brito, S. A., & Viding, E. (2011). The impact of child maltreatment: A review of neurobiological and genetic factors, *Frontiers in Psychiatry*, 2: 48.

National Scientific Council on the Developing Child. (2020). Connecting the brain to the rest of the body: Early childhood development and lifelong health are deeply intertwined. Working paper no. 15. http://developingchild.harvard.edu/wp-content/uploads/2020/06/wp15_health_FINAL_061520.pdf.

Nermeen, E., Nokali, E., Bachman, H. J., & Votruba-Drzal, E. (2010). Parent's involvement and children's academic and social development in elementary school. *Child Development*, 81(3), 988–1005.

Ochsner, K. N., & Gross, J. J. (2005). The cognitive control of emotion, *Trends in Cognitive Sciences*, 9(5), 242–249.

Ohly, H., White, M., & Wheeler, B. (2016). Attention Restoration Theory: A systematic review of the attention restoration potential of exposure to natural environments. *Journal of Toxicology and Environmental Health – Part B: Critical Reviews.* https://doi.org/10.1080/10937404.2016.1196155.

Panksepp, J. (1998). Attention deficit hyperactivity disorders, psychostimulants, and intolerance of childhood playfulness: A tragedy in the making? *Current Directions in Psychological Science* 7 (3), 91–98.

Perry, B. (1997). Incubated in terror: neurodevelopmental factors in the cycle of violence. In J. Osofsky (Ed.), *Children, youth and violence: The search for solutions* (pp. 124–148). New York: Guilford Press.

Pfeiffer, S. I., & Petscher, Y. (2008). Identifying young, gifted children using the gifted rating scales: Preschool/kindergarten form. *Gifted Child Quarterly*, 52(1). https://journals.sagepub.com/doi/10.1177/0016986207311055.

Plucker, J., & Barab, S. A. (2005). The importance of contexts in theories of giftedness: learning to embrace the messy joys of subjectivity. In R. J. Sternberg & J. E. Davidson (Eds.), *Conceptions of giftedness* (pp. 201–216). Cambridge: Cambridge University Press.

Pollak, S. D., Cicchetti, D., Hornuny, K., & Reed, A. (2000). Recognizing emotion in faces: Developmental effects of child abuse and neglect. *Developmental Psychology*, 36, 679–688.

Rathunde, K., & Csikszentmihalyi, M. (2006). The developing person: An experiential perspective. In W. Damon & R. M. Lerner (Eds.), *Handbook of child psychology: Theoretical models of human development*, vol. I (pp. 465–515). Hoboken, NJ: Wiley & Sons.

Renzulli, J. S. (1978). What makes giftedness? Re-examining a definition. *Phi Delta Kappan* 60(3), 180–184.

Renzulli, J. S. (2019). A practical system for identifying gifted and talented students. In J. T. Pardeck & J. W. Murphy (Eds.), *Young gifted children: Identification, programming and socio-psychological issues* (pp. 9–18). Abingdon and New York: Routledge.

Renzulli, J. S., & Reis, S. M. (2018). The three-ring conception of giftedness: A developmental approach for promoting creative productivity in young people. In S. I. Pfeiffer (Ed.), *APA handbook of giftedness and talent* (pp. 185–200). Washington, DC: American Psychological Association.

Ritzi, R. M., & Ray, D. C. (2017). Intensive short-term child-centred play therapy and externalising behaviours in children. *International Journal of Play Therapy*, 26(1), 33–46.

Robinson, C., & Brown, A. M. (2016). Considering sensory processing issues in trauma affected children: The physical environment in children's residential homes. *Scottish Journal of Residential Childcare*, 15(1).

Roedell, W. C. (1989). Early development of gifted children. In J. Van Tassel-Basja & P. Olszewski-Kublius (Eds.), *Patterns of influence on gifted learners, the home, the self and the school* (pp. 13–28). New York: Teachers College Press.

Roedell, W. C. (1984). Vulnerabilities of highly gifted children. *Roeper Review*, 6(3), 127–130.

Roisman, G. I., Padron, E., Sroufe, L. A., & Egeland, B. (2002). Earned–secure attachment status in retrospect and prospect. *Child Development*, 73 (4), 1204–1219.

Runco, M. A. (1991). Dimensions of divergent thinkers. In *Divergent thinking* (pp. 87–134). Norwood, NJ: Ablex.

Ruskin, E. M., Kasari, C., Mundy, P. & Sigman, M. (1994). Attention to people and toys during social and object mastery in children with Down syndrome. *American Journal on Mental Retardation*, 99, 103–111.

Scottish Government. (2010). *Pre-birth to three: Positive outcomes for Scotland's children and families.* Edinburgh: Scottish Government.

Siegel, D. (2003). An interpersonal neurobiology of psychotherapy: The developing mind and the resolution of trauma. In M. F. Solomon & D. J. Siegel (Eds.), *Healing trauma: Attachment, mind, body, and brain.* London: W. W. Norton & Company.

Stern, D. N. (1998). *The interpersonal world of the infant: A view from psychoanalysis and developmental psychology.* London: Karnac.

Thelen, E., & Smith, L. B. (2006). Dynamic systems theory. In W. Damon & R. Lerner (Eds.), *Handbook of child psychology*, vol. I (pp. 258–312). Hoboken, NJ: John Wiley & Sons.

Vaivre-Douret, L. (2011). Developmental and cognitive characteristics of "high-level potentialities" (highly gifted) children. *International Journal of Paediatrics, 1687–9740*, 420297.

Whitters, H. G. (2019). *Attainment and executive functioning in the early years.* Abingdon and New York: Routledge.

Zhou, M., & Brown, D. (2015). *Educational learning theories*, 2nd edition, Education Open Textbooks, 1. https://oer.galileo.usg.edu/education-textbooks/1.

6   Research, theory, and intervention

The final chapter describes a human being as an evolving bio-psychological organism. Proximal processes, dispositions, and structuring proclivities contribute to an infant's understanding of his interactions. Traits and behaviours are contextualised through reference to the social address model (Magnusson & Stattin, 2006). This model presents the principles of novelty, pleasure, and reality in a context of learning opportunities. The model promotes comprehension of each person's unique interpretation of and reaction to an environment which is influenced by his or her perception of variants. The play cycle is reviewed in this chapter and play flow considered. Inclusive pedagogy must include opportunities for children of low and high abilities and many different stages in between.

This chapter concludes with implications for the future. Current messages from research, policy, and practice identify a two-pronged approach as the way forward by supporting individual attainment and by improving access to education, health care, and income. Findings by Tal (2021) highlighted four main influences upon development as agency, relationships, education, and professional expertise. A core competency which is required by a professional is knowledge and understanding of infant mental health (Association of Infant Mental Health UK, 2021).

Attachment over time

In 2020, the National Scientific Council on the Developing Child (2020) published information to inform the creation of a foundation for health and development. Research indicated significant stages of development that pertained to the pre-birth months and the earliest years of childhood. These findings are reminiscent of sensitive periods for learning as previously highlighted by John Bowlby (1997).

Brain architecture is affected by internal and external influences such as interaction of genes and experiences over time. The report by the National Scientific Council on the Developing Child (2020) describes interdependency between human systems. For example, a context of feedback loops are used to send signals from the brain to influence responses by the heart and lungs,

DOI: 10.4324/9781003358107-6

digestive system, energy production, infection control, and physical growth. The learning environment affects brain development, which directs actions and reactions in the physiological systems. Default patterns of response are acquired in the earliest years and activated throughout our lifespans.

Homeostasis refers to a balance of the systems within this operation. Adaptation to threat is termed "allostasis". If the body's reaction to a stressful situation is prolonged, for example raised blood pressure and rapid heartbeat, then long-term damage may occur. The developing pattern of responses can include a propensity to negative reaction. Consequently, the period between an individual encountering stressful circumstances and a physiological reaction by the body's systems may shorten over time and be disproportionate to the context.

Comprehending, and responding to, relationality of physical and mental health is key to supporting attainment. Current messages from policy and practice are equally applicable to all children regardless of ability or short- and long-term additional support for learning needs. A two-pronged approach is the way forward by supporting individual attainment *and* by improving access to education, health care, and income. Responsive actions include the creation of relationships with primary carers and peers, reducing family sources of stress in addition to a child's personal stress, and, finally, strengthening skills, which provide a necessary baseline for self-regulation and executive functioning (National Scientific Council on the Developing Child, 2020).

Sensitive responding is based upon the features of attachment theory (Simpson & Belsky, 2008), and interventions are developed from this rich source of knowledge and understanding. Three particular aspects of this theory are the synchronisation of parent–infant behaviour in the post-birth stages, the young child's need, and his tendency to seek proximity to the primary carer, and the pathway to learning which is created as the attachment relationship matures and changes.

At the moment of birth, a mother experiences hormonal influences that support her to bond with the new baby. Exaggerated facial expressions, slow and intentional speech, and seeking out close eye and facial contact are natural behaviours from a new mother towards her infant. The infant responds by engaging in three types of behaviour that support *his* need to have contact (Simpson & Belsky, 2008).

1   The baby will use signalling to indicate his desire for positive interaction, rooting for milk, seeking his mother's eye contact or being still as he listens and senses his mother in the early stages post-birth.
2   He will use aversive behaviours, for example, crying and screaming, to prompt his carer to respond to his needs.
3   Over time, the infant will use active intentional behaviours and move towards his attachment figure.

Bowlby (1997) commented that lack of response by a carer can cause a fourth behaviour which encompasses withdrawal, silence, and despondency.

These survival strategies result from a lack of safety provided by a primary carer as the baby attempts to hide from perceived threat and danger.

The interpretation of the first relationships in life for a baby are retained within an inner working model. This experience represents a blueprint model of self and others within attachment dyads. The function of the model is integral to the child's understanding of future relationships with peers and potential lifelong partners (Bretherton & Munholland, 2008). The attachment working model is relationship-specific, and it is influenced within numerous daily interactions between the young child and primary figures.

Mikulincer and Shaver (2008) applied the term "broaden and build the cycle of attachment security" in a specific context of emotional development and well-being of insecurely attached adults. These authors promoted the use of actual or symbolic representations of attachment figures to instil self-worth associated with positive relational experiences. Photographs of family members or partners are common screensavers on phones or computers. Activating secure attachment status through mental representations of personal value to a child or adult induces the effects experienced within these responsive relationships. Over time, coping skills will be activated autonomously and lead to the operation of other behavioural systems, for example, exploration and caregiving. Psychological benefits pertain to reduction of distress and restoration of emotional stability.

Aspects of attachment were studied by Mikulincer and Shaver (2008) in a context of adult participants. Results highlighted outcomes that inform interventions for children in their early years and provide a rationale for practice. The first aspect refers to life appraisal which encompasses an ability to assess negative situations and to maintain optimism, hope, and a sense of control. The second aspect relates to mental representations of others, which includes the belief that other people have positive intentions. The research included participants who were partners, and findings showed that activating positive mental representations of a partner, even momentarily, promoted positive expectations about his or her behaviour.

Mikulincer and Shaver (2008) applied the term "authentic self-esteem" to describe the third aspect as confidence in one's worthiness, competence, and mastery of a situation. These authors indicated that this aspect has the potential to engender autonomous emotion regulation which can reduce stress, even if the attachment figure is unavailable. The experience of being loved and valued by an attachment person can lead to a personal mental representation of self in this context. The final aspect is termed "constructive coping strategies", which encompasses the ability to minimise stress through the use of problem-solving, planning, applying cognition skills, and accessing support from others.

Gross (1999) described these types of strategies as "antecedent-focused emotion regulation". This concept referred to minimisation of emotions prior to the full negative effects being experienced. Thirty years ago, Lazarus (1991) described the same process as a "short circuit of threat". This term referred to the ability of an individual to use the functional and adaptive qualities of emotions instead of being affected adversely by dysfunctional aspects. Secure attachment supports a person to express distress, to verbalise experiences, to seek help from an appropriate source, and, finally, to implement effective coping strategies that minimise the impact of negative emotions.

Inner working models evolve through adaptation to changing circumstances and relationships. A primary carer will inevitably have lapses in sensitivity which can relate to issues such as a carer's illness, prioritisation of tasks, short-term distractions, or protecting the young child from immediate danger. Stability in the attachment relationship is maintained by the child accepting these short-term lapses and the carer being aware of the need to repair the relationship over time. It is felt that children are more likely to develop adaptive working models if parents encourage a child to explore his inner world and to communicate emotions (Bretherton & Munholland, 2008). The need for self-protection can also influence a child's rejection of a relationship in response to interpretation and adaptation of circumstances and actions by the adult.

The secure relationship supports a baby to mature into a competent emotionally aware child who has a set of skills to use in self-regulation of emotions and behaviour. Research links secure attachment to an increase in the child's emotional understanding of self and others, to social cognition and formation of peer relationships, memory, and, finally, to the development of conscience in the early years (Thompson, 2008). Memory is influenced by representation of emotions associated with attachment-related events, and conscience is linked to compliance and cooperation within the dyadic relationship of a primary carer.

Mikulincer and Shaver (2008) also referred to memory, and their research findings indicated that preconscious activation of the attachment system increased access to mental representation of an attachment figure. The study described how these mental processes could influence intentions and behaviour prior to conscious formulation. The dispositional attachment style is informed by experiences, for example, positive expectations, and a route to gaining support. Even young babies can use help-seeking behaviours which are directed towards their secure attachment figure, and in adulthood sources of support are easily identified and accessed confidently. The negative experiences that lead to insecure attachment can cause children and adults to use secondary survival strategies, for example, hyperactivation or deactivation of the attachment system (Mikulincer & Shaver, 2008).

Person–environment interaction

Bronfenbrenner (2005) explored the theory of human development, and he proposed that family was the most significant influence in the earliest years and impactful throughout adult life. According to Bronfenbrenner, family is defined as a group of people who have unconditional commitment to one another's well-being. It is useful to read this theorist's views from a practitioner's perspective. Bronfenbrenner focused upon the operational aspects of the parent–child dyad and influence from a third party. He describes the third party as composed of friends, community, or organisations that facilitate optimum effect from the two-person system of parent and child. In working with families over many years, I have found that each parent–child dyad has a distinct identity which is steeped in a family culture influenced by historical and current experiences. The dyad evolves over time, and the relationship has immense potential to support development of the two members: parent and child.

In a recent publication, Nagy and Nagy (2022) refer to the skilful adaptation of working conditions within a context of the COVID-19 pandemic in Hungary. During lockdown periods, role-modelling of physical and emotional nurturing by early years practitioners was replaced by the use of information technology. This medium provided an aid to maintain communication between services and home. Key workers used the format of Facebook to upload videos of activities that promoted parent–child interaction within the home environment, and it supported the family's processing of trauma associated with the pandemic. This study highlighted the ingenuity of practitioners in responding to the unprecedented crisis of COVID-19 in addition to the importance of person-to-person interactions.

Research by Duffy et al. (2021) investigated the use of a screening tool for the long-term mental-health condition of post-traumatic stress disorder (PTSD). The participant group was 141 young people who had experienced maltreatment in childhood. Findings indicated three items which were associated with PTSD as a history of being on the child-protection register, prior mental-health issues, and interpersonal trauma. These authors reported an unexpected finding as data from the young people that identified the death or loss of a close relationship as a traumatic experience. This research indicates the importance of interpersonal relationships to reduce the impact of loss.

Tal (2021) recently highlighted four main influential concepts upon development.

1   The child's agency.
2   Interactions and relationships.
3   Educational practice.
4   Professional development.

Agency refers to the child's ability and capacity to influence operations within daily living. Ryecraft (2019) reviewed research on the agency of children who were living within a disadvantaged context but deemed to have higher than average ability. The findings identified 16 common traits. It is interesting that the single trait that negatively affected attainment related to limited communication skills, and it is described within the research as a low level of knowledge and vocabulary. The development of verbal communication commences in the home environment, from birth, and the aforementioned research highlights the need for children and families to be supported in their earliest years.

The traits from the research by Ryecraft (2019) are regarded as positive influences upon a child's agency, his ability to embrace learning opportunities, and his achievement of potential. Findings indicated the 15 positive traits as the child being alert and curious, independent, using non-verbal fluency, being an experiential learner, and creative, able to take risks, and to demonstrate a sense of humour, the use of imagery in language, showing leadership skills, interested in music and art, responsible, adaptable, externally motivated, using memory and observational skills, and being responsive to learning.

A research study by Zero to Three (2017) publicised behaviours that could indicate concerns regarding an infant or young child's mental health in the earliest years. The research findings included: chronic eating or sleeping difficulties, irritability, difficult to console with excessive crying, clear distress if primary carer leaves, difficulty in adapting to new situations, easily startled by familiar routines, inability to establish relationships with other children or adults, excessive hitting, biting, and pushing of other children or very withdrawn behaviour, little to no emotion, engaging compulsive activities, excessive and repeated tantrums/aggressive behaviours, little interest in social interaction, immature communication, and indicative loss of earlier developmental achievements. The works by Ryecraft (2019) and Zero to Three (2017) present broad lists of behaviours associated with attainment or mental health. Each child's interpretation of and reaction to influences is unique, and responses should reflect personal characteristics, and emotional effect.

Social address model

These traits and behaviours can be understood in greater depth by reference to the social address model by Magnusson and Stattin (2006). This theoretical model presents the principles of novelty, pleasure, and reality in a context of an infant, child, or adult embracing learning opportunities. The social address model promotes comprehension of each person's unique interpretation and reaction to an environment which is based upon his or her perceptions of variants. The research is informative to educators as all children should be supported to develop these positive traits in the early years to promote development. Therapeutic approaches have been introduced to early years work in the past decade within contexts of targeted intervention and generic pedagogy. Organisations that specialise in working with families focus upon nurturing secure attachment between parent and child primarily and subsequent relationships thereafter.

Intervention strategies

In a context of infant mental health, the attachment relationship from child to adult, and the bonding relationship from adult to child, are key aspects of healthy development and resilience to adversities. Barlow (2016) described several factors of significance to the strengthening of an attachment bond based upon the principles by Simpson and Belsky (2008): a parent's sensitivity to an infant's needs and emotional reactions, the quality of attunement from parent to infant, and parental ability to reflect and adapt behaviour to an infant's presentation, and interactions within a midrange context. In curricular guidance, the term "sensitive responding" is often used to promote the behaviour, emotion, and intent of an adult's reflective interaction to an infant's needs and preferences.

Berlin et al. (2008) identified three approaches that could accumulatively respond to attachment needs of infants. The three approaches are interdependent and incorporated into many formal and informal intervention contexts:

1   First, implementation of intervention that targets a process of change in the parent's internal working model by prompting reflection, and re-evaluation of parenting skills.
2   Second, the creation of a base of knowledge which can be used to change a parent's behaviour towards an infant by supporting interpretation of the infant's needs and interests.
3   Third, the development of a therapeutic alliance between professional and parent as an effective medium to promote learning and development of parent and child.

A recent report from Child Protection Committees in Scotland (Scottish Government, 2021) identifies key approaches to minimising the impact of neglect: clarify the issues, engage the family, create a safe environment, increase parenting sensitivity, assess family circumstances, support parenting capacity to change, and reflect upon historical family circumstances. This report is designed to provide guidance to services and advocates implementation of a comprehensive, multilayered response. Time and timeliness for change and development are highlighted alongside an approach that addresses social supports and inclusion. This approach ensures that vulnerable families receive help that is equitable, proportionate, and effective.

Family programmes from birth, and even the pre-birth period, can provide valuable planned and spontaneous opportunities for learning. A literature search by Hogg (2019) identified 27 specialised parent–infant teams throughout the United Kingdom that provide intensive support to vulnerable mothers and babies during the perinatal period, pre-birth to one year. These multidisciplinary teams promote secure attachment between parent and infant by using a therapeutic approach. Ultimately, each child requires a consistently secure relationship with a carer to support activation of curiosity and exploration and to kindle a desire for knowledge. Nurture groups and nurturing practices are recognised as impactful upon social and emotional competencies in the early years and primary-school settings, and as contributing to closing the attainment gap.

Doyle and Cicchetti (2017) conducted a broad literature review on attachment, and the discussion highlighted findings from the Bucharest Early Intervention Project. The study encompassed development of children who had been placed in Romanian orphanages at birth. Findings indicated that the children had ongoing developmental deficiencies across all domains. The study acknowledged that neural plasticity and intervention can support the negative effects to be reduced in some children. However, a significant finding indicated that mental representations from early experiences have the potential to influence parent–child relationships in subsequent generations. Maladaptive parenting requires intervention beyond parenting programmes, and these authors refer to the use of child–parent psychotherapy. Child–parent psychotherapy is founded upon the parent and child dyad being regarded as the client rather than separate individuals. Responsive intervention focuses upon safety, affect regulation and the creation of a shared trauma narrative.

Theory of development

Bronfenbrenner (2005) investigated the concept of developmental outcomes and explored the establishment of mental processes. Developmental outcomes occur from the joint functioning of a person and his proximal or distal environment. There are many similarities among the neural workings of human beings; however, the importance of personal characteristics upon subjective interpretation, and actions, was consistently promoted by Bronfenbrenner. This theorist described changes that occur in the development of a person between systems as ecological transitions (Bronfenbrenner, 1979). Influences that prompt these changes are known as "variable factors".

Patterns of motivation and actions create developmental trajectories which can be observed within different settings, for example, home or nursery, indoor or outdoor play. The trans-contextual dyad of adult and child supports transference of knowledge and application within different circumstances. Bronfenbrenner (2005) applied the term "mesosystem phenomenon" as the changes gained developmental validity by occurring in more than one setting. A secure attachment relationship is a key influence upon this event of ecological transitioning. Bronfenbrenner indicated that momentum gave meaning and perpetuity to short-term molecular behaviours which were categorised as stimulus-responses or transitory actions. These behaviours subsequently transformed into longer-term molar activities if the conditions were conducive.

Bronfenbrenner (2005) researched the concept of variance. He believed that variance between human beings related to a heritability system. This means that genetic influences are actualised into observable phenomena. In the context of an early years nursery, a practitioner conducts daily observations on key children, and she rapidly accumulates examples of influences upon the child's functioning although evidence of a genetic link is unconfirmed. Variation is demonstrated by joint functioning of proximal processes and characteristics. The child's actions are influenced by his personality and specific strengths or weaknesses. Practitioners are well aware of variance through observing different actions, behaviour, and emotional reactions from siblings to the same family circumstances, and to their involvement with the learning environment of a playroom.

Influences may be formative life events or the predispositions which are based upon personal characteristics of the individual. Examples are genetic defects, congenital damage, severe and long-term illness, in addition to a high level of ability, and capacity which is built upon good health at birth, genetic potential, and learning opportunities. A change in mental health can be the result of these issues, and this is regarded as a triggering event to alteration of the child or parent's interpretation, perceptions, and reaction to a proximal environment. Bronfenbrenner (2005) termed the outcome of these developmental processes as having a social stimulus value, and his work continues to increase comprehension of negative and positive influences which are relevant to today's society.

Bronfenbrenner and Morris (2006) explored indirect impact from a deficiency, for example, a low birthweight that could reduce a child's capacity to engage with learning. Low birthweight can be associated with many adverse childhood experiences, including poverty and poor health of the mother. Research has also indicated that stress exhibited by a baby in adverse circumstances will result in a stress response by a parent whereas a baby who demonstrates increasing competence and social skills will prompt a parent to provide stimulation and lead to reciprocal interaction. Parenting work with primary carers and their children is a relevant and valuable response to these issues.

Clemens et al. (2020) recently conducted research on an extensive sample group of over 2,000 parents in Germany. The results showed that parents who had experienced adverse childhood experiences exhibited a higher acceptance of negative behaviours in their own parenting roles. This study focused specifically upon behaviours which had resulted in a head trauma upon the child. Findings indicated that a mother's resilience to a crying baby might be reduced if her personal memory of childhood stress was associated with negative responses from her own parents. Memories retained from early childhood experiences shape interactions between adults and children within each generation.

Therapeutic alliance

Cain (2010) noted that the skill of a third party could facilitate development of others, and he promoted the therapeutic relationship as an effective medium for communication. Twenty years previously, Carl Rogers indicated one such skill as the ability to enter the perceptual world of a child, and he applied the term "therapeutic alliance" (Rogers, 1990). The Scottish Government (2009) describe this alliance as contributing to a healing process within the body and mind of parents and children. Hope and potential for change are key messages gained from research on these topics.

Several authors have studied the therapeutic relationship in a context of parenting support. An extensive literature review was conducted by Moran and a research team in 2004, and it projected an important message in response to issues that affected the capacity and motivation of a carer to engage with parenting support (Moran et al., 2004). The use of relational skills to engage parents was a common factor that featured in the findings of this review. A previous study by Benjamin and Karpiak (2001) had indicated that this type of relationship also had a positive effect upon personality stabilisation. Braun et al. (2006) commented that the therapeutic alliance could be used by a parent to activate support from a professional in response to current and potential needs which were forecast.

Carl Rogers (1990) studied in the field of psychotherapy, but parallels can be drawn with his findings to the professional–parent relationship in the early years sector. Rogers identified six necessary conditions to the creation of an alliance between professional and a client (Whitters, 2015).

1   Two human beings, a therapist and a client, who are in psychological contact. For example, a practitioner and parent communicating about needs and support.
2   The client existing in a state of incongruence. For example, a parent experiencing mental health issues within a chaotic lifestyle.
3   The therapist existing in a state of congruence and integrated in the relationship. For example, a practitioner demonstrating empathy and supporting containment in this context.
4   The therapist experiences unconditional positive regard for the client. For example, the practitioner demonstrates a caring and non-judgemental approach.
5   The therapist experiences an empathic understanding of the client's frame of reference and attempts to communicate this understanding. For example, the practitioner uses tracking and description to emphasise care and understanding.
6   The therapist achieves a positive communication of empathic understanding and unconditional positive regard to a minimal level. For example, an effective communication medium is achieved within a therapeutic alliance.

Professionals can achieve congruence through self-disclosure, articulation of thoughts and emotions, and responses which are not necessarily bound by specific requirements of a professional discipline (Klein et al., 2002). The effect of congruence can be transferred within the medium of a relationship, and Rogers promoted this stage as significant to creation of a therapeutic alliance. Rogers (1990) applied the term "transcendent phenomenon" to describe the effect of congruence upon a client that encompasses transfer of emotional, physical, and social well-being from service-provider to service-user. The term "value system" was linked to this alliance, and Rogers indicated that the inner choices of a parent had greater value than choices of compliance within the relationship. It is important that the developing person, the parent, is aware of undergoing this process of change and placing value and worth upon her progress. The parent's comprehension of self will alter over time, and past perceptions of the world are actively rejected as new interpretation emerges.

Cain (2010) had expressed that secure attachment and corrective relational experiences had a positive impact upon the congruence of parent and professional. The therapeutic alliance is a fluctuating and ongoing medium for communication which has great potential impact upon learning and development. The relationship may be fragile in the earliest stages, but it can be consolidated and strengthened over time. Consistency and predictability of reaction and actions from the attachment figure are key outcomes from a secure relationship.

Theories provide understanding, and direction, to the implementation of interventions that target change and development of parenting skills. Lave and Wenger (1991) described the process by which a parent integrates within an established socio-cultural practice. For example, participating in formal and informal parenting intervention within the context of a service-pedagogy. Parental choice, empowerment, decision-making, and personality stabilisation are aspects of many parenting programmes and interventions. Over time, the parent adopts the socio-cultural approaches and becomes an agent of practice within this context. Convergence and agreement in the perceptions of professionals and parents have been linked to positive outcomes in contexts of child protection cases (Cleaver & Freeman, 1995; Trotter, 2002).

Resources, disposition, and demand characteristics

The development of human beings follows a pattern that commences with a young baby's predisposition to focus upon his physical and social environment, and, ultimately, his representation within these contexts. Babies respond to vestibular stimulation by reacting to the physical responses of different people, and newborn babies will start to demonstrate preferences in the earliest days of life. Every new parent quickly learns to interpret her baby's cues of likes or dislikes in relation to physical interaction. Some babies prefer to be held in a prone position, feeling the warmth of an adult's arms, or facing the primary carer and absorbing voice and smell, or in the vertical position to look outwards and view the wider world.

A human being is an evolving bio-psychological organism. Proximal processes are regular, and reciprocal interactions occur between a person and others, objects, or communication systems. These processes are regarded as developmental, and improvement in the quality leads to a higher level of heritability and elevated developmental functioning (Bronfenbrenner, 2005; Whitters, 2015). Dispositions relate to personal interests which can activate proximal processes. Bronfenbrenner and Morris (2006) used the term "structuring proclivities" to describe a baby's inclination to seek out particular proximal processes and to develop and sustain reciprocal interactions. Over time, the young child begins to gain an understanding of his interactions which pertain to deeper conceptual levels as maturity increases.

Demand characteristics refer to the motivation and needs of an individual which can support or can prevent proximal processing. Bronfenbrenner and Morris (2006) made a distinction between developmentally generative characteristics and developmentally disruptive characteristics (Whitters, 2015).

1. Developmentally generative characteristics: Proximal processes have greater power to support actualisation of genetic potential within a consistent and positive living environment and lifestyle.

2. Developmentally disruptive characteristics: Proximal processes in a disadvantaged context will hinder development potential. Disadvantage is categorised as instability in the domains of space and time. This negative influence is represented by chaotic and unpredictable lifestyles within non-stimulating and disorganised households.

The findings by Moran et al. (2004) on early years provision described the organisation of an environment as a determinant factor in the functioning of processes as an asset or deterrent to development. An environment functions and changes through ongoing processes of interaction and interdependence in respect of social, cultural, and physical factors (Magnusson & Stattin, 2006). In early years services, the presentation of a learning environment is determined by health and safety parameters, curricular guidance, and the unique pedagogy of each organisation in addition to practitioner skill and creativity.

Thelen and Smith (2006) applied the terms "coupling" and "continuity" in order to promote further comprehension of developmental influences. Coupling refers to links and interactions between all components within each person's developing system. Continuity indicates that processes are iterative and always based upon the merging of previous and current experiences. The parent and professional are key to supporting activation of these processes in the context of a child's development. Proximal processing may extend over time if there are influences or characteristics from more than one source. Educators and parents are distinctive influential sources of learning for children, and the home environment may also be enriched by input from siblings, grandparents, and the local community. A context of multiple rich influences increases retention of learning. A positive learning environment can be gained through attendance at an early years service and primary school, which includes home–school links.

Each person is an active intentional component within a complex, dynamic, person-environment system (Bronfenbrenner, 2005). As an inexperienced practitioner, I felt challenged by this statement, and I sought understanding by focusing upon my practical base of knowledge, which was gained from implementation in the field. I realised that this research finding matched my daily experiences in the playrooms, and it granted worthiness to the daily interactions of the early years workforce. Every infant, parent, and practitioner actively contributes to changing an environment and creating learning opportunities that instil knowledge and understanding within each person. The person and the environment are interdependent and contribute to development of the system, the individual, and the local setting.

In 2006, Spencer contributed to this debate through her research within an African American context. This researcher indicated that differences in perceptions could account for human variation in the context of development (Spencer, 2006). This approach is known as the phenomenological variant of the ecological systems model. Differentiation, and interaction of resources, disposition, and demand characteristics, can account for variation of actions by human beings to the same circumstances. It is often the case that several siblings display different reactions to their shared home micro-system. It is important to note that differentiation and interaction also affect the primary carer who is a separate, but influential entity to the child.

Focus of attention and practice

Bronfenbrenner and Morris (2006) commented that the power of the bio-ecological model to affect a child's development increases in accordance with the focus of attention by the developing child and the parent. The focus of attention within a parent–child dyad can be supported and promoted through intervention by a third party. The third party relates to practitioners, therapists, or any influential beings. Demand characteristics from a help-seeking parent can also intensify the focus of attention.

These theories are relevant to strategic and operational practice in services today. The current approach to family support is tailoring intervention in accordance with family perceptions of need, characteristics, strengths, and specific areas identified for development within a context of child protection. Establishing patterns of positive parent and child interaction can be linked to a third party. In current services, an early years worker, health visitor, speech therapist, social worker, or educational psychologist promote the agency of a parent–child dyad. This third party supports agency by giving recognition to the parent's role which strengthens, consolidates, and highlights the significance of influences. The professional directly supports the development of the parent's skills in order to actualise potential of the child. Bronfenbrenner (2005) also placed importance on informal and indirect third-person influences from family and community throughout daily living.

Ten years ago, research by Walsh et al. (2010) identified four principles for implementing a curriculum in a specific context of children who demonstrated higher than average ability. These principles are still applicable and current to education in early years settings, regardless of the child's ability in relation to a norm:

1   Identification of child's ability through practitioner observation and information from parents. This information informs the creation of an individual learning plan that reflects developmental needs, interests, and personality of the child.

2   Presentation of a child-led learning environment which is based upon children's interests and a pedagogy that incorporates opportunities for accelerated content through scaffolding by practitioners.

3   Lateral enrichment opportunities that feature in the layout of an environment and support children to make choices and to link concepts throughout a playroom and outdoor play spaces.

4   Peer interaction between children of similar ability by mixing different age groups and encouraging parents to present stimulating social opportunities for sibling play at home and peers in the community.

Enrichment, extension, and differentiation

Knowledge and understanding of developmental goals which are based upon the norms for an age range inform the creation and delivery of a curriculum within a year group. This pedagogy can reflect the needs of many children, and knowledge of norms is a foundation of early years practice. However, the ability to recognise and to respond to a child's potential which is above or below these developmental levels are also essential skills in a context of inclusion and equality. Enrichment tends to be the approach that has prevailed in education as a strategy to support developmental potential.

Enrichment of learning opportunities reflects a child's interests and schemas at any point in time and leads to a deeper detailed level of understanding of a topic beyond mandatory curricular content. Extension of an activity can incorporate opportunities for divergent thinking and creativity. Extension invariably leads to enrichment due to activation of the child's curiosity and motivation to satisfy his desire for knowledge and understanding.

Differentiation of pedagogy in the delivery of curricular content can take many forms. Taylor (2019) analysed the responses of 5,000 teachers and identified five common aspects of practice. This study had been conducted in a context of primary schooling; however, these five classroom strategies can also be applied within an early years setting and home environment:

1   **Oral questions**: The use of open questions, prompts, and probes to further the child's knowledge and to support comprehension by tailoring interactions to suit current capacity and ability.

2   **Feedback**: The provision of feedback that responds to each child's output can provide scaffolding of knowledge in verbal format, and it builds upon the current base of information which is held by a child.

3   **Linking with prior attainment**: This strategy supports a child to recognise, and to use his current base of knowledge and understanding to advance to the next level. Learning follows an iterative pathway in response to the child's ability.

4   **Scaffolding**: An effective and common practice throughout many different learning environments that requires an adult or peer to use encouragement, specific ideas, role-modelling, prompts, and probes, and to demonstrate an interest in the child's interests to further development.

5   **Outcome**: It may be necessary to have a range of outcomes for children who present at different stages of development. This approach requires an educator to consider each task as composed of many aspects and to determine appropriate goals/outcomes which can reflect every child's capacity, ability, and recognise attainment.

A catalyst for learning is the secure relationship between child and a supportive adult. Good mental health empowers the young child to seek out opportunities, to make effective social choices, and to gain satisfaction and fulfilment from furthering knowledge and understanding. The home environment presents a rich cultural experience for learning within a family unit. It is a venue in which children can observe and adopt values, attitudes, and beliefs of parents and gain opportunities for accelerated and enriched learning with older siblings. Supporting children in the home environment does not need to entail formal educational experiences, but parents, brothers, and sisters can utilise everyday resources to activate intrinsic motivation in a child.

Box 6.1 Example from practice

Cold rain slides down the windows in straight lines, and it splashes loudly onto the white painted windowsills. Three-year-old Gracey and her older sister, Brooke, are standing side by side as they observe the watery scene outside. Gracey sighs as she brushes her fine red hair away from her eyes and looks toward her sister, expectantly. The world is experiencing lengthy periods of society lockdown to temper the virulence of COVID-19. Home-schooling, home-friendships, and home-play are familiar concepts to every child and parent. Brooke turns her mind to entertainment and places a pink spiral notebook on the low glass coffee table alongside several little coloured pencils. For the next ten minutes, the 7-year-old proceeds to teach her little sister ante-preschool and preschool skills. She is inadvertently scaffolding Gracey's development during play. Their secure sibling relationship ensures that Gracey invests in the tuition which is freely given by her sister. The skill set acquired by the 3-year-old is multifold:

- Using fine motor skills and hand–eye coordination to pick up a pencil from the slippery table surface.
- Observing and copying the role model of Brooke's adept finger movements to position a pencil for creativity.
- Understanding and reproducing hard and soft strokes, noticing light and shade as she strives to copy the numbers and kisses that Brooke instigates upon the page.
- Coordinating her little hand and wrist to reproduce the circles of sunshine one way and the other, her wrist action gaining skill and speed over time.

- Moving each pencil up and down, little ticks and big ticks, filling each white page.
- Selecting a sheet of paper, listening, and counting as she follows the noise of the spiral notebook releasing a page, hole by hole.
- Folding the paper along its faint printed lines, using both hands as tools, a firm press and creativity is activated in the 3-year-old explorer.

The early stages of literacy are fun to learn in a play environment and gained easily within the context of a positive sibling relationship on a rainy, lockdown Saturday afternoon at home.

Learning environments should promote intrinsic rather than extrinsic reward and activate the child's curiosity and motivation to learn within a cultural context. Creativity should be embraced and used to forge links between areas of learning. Diversity should be celebrated in order to recognise unique attributes as positive.

Knowledge and understanding

One key aspect of learning involves delivery of knowledge in a manner and medium that promotes understanding by each recipient. Instruction needs to be on par with the developmental level of the individual child and to be accompanied by motivational prompts that match his personality, needs, and interests at a point in time. Traditional programmes such as heuristic play are useful for the newly ambulant child (Whitters, 2017). This specially prepared play environment can support young children to follow their interests and to learn incrementally as the experience is offered twice weekly. A range of toys is presented to the child that support problem-solving, sensory exploration, and imaginative play. A multitude of containers support schemas and activate the child's interest in developing the play environment. The key worker responds to the child's emotional and social needs within this context, which increases the child's capacity to seek out learning opportunities independently. The quiet atmosphere is conducive to good mental health and exploration.

The term "observational learning" refers to a child observing a scene, interpreting the actions of peers or adults, and subsequently reproducing his acquired knowledge in the same context or another. An early years setting, or home environment, can provide multiple opportunities to support observational learning. Researchers identified four coexisting processes that occur within this context (Zhou & Brown, 2015):

1   **Attention**: The child will demonstrate a capacity to focus upon one activity and minimise the effect from other influences.
2   **Retention**: The child will create memories from his exploration which increase his comprehension.

3 **Production**: The child will apply his knowledge to current and future activities.
4 **Motivation**: The child will demonstrate intrinsic motivation, which links to his curiosity and interests.

A child requires a broad understanding of the world – not just facts and information, but many opportunities to experience and to apply what he has learned in practice. The young learner will use objects in different ways and gain understanding of concepts such as size, weight, height, and length. Most nurseries set up defined areas of play which are designed to promote contextual experiences within a playroom, for example, a home corner, book corner, an arts and crafts area, a cognitive area, and physical play. A child can independently extend his learning by linking adjacent toys and materials in response to interests and needs and to create something new and personal. Inclusive pedagogy must include opportunities for children of low and high abilities and many different stages in-between. Responsive staff can nurture positive relationships and provide rich opportunities to support formation of a child's neural connections.

During the first wave of the COVID-19 pandemic, children in UK nurseries were restricted to several small groups called bubbles (Early Learning and Childcare Directorate, 2020). The rationale for these circumstances was based upon necessity for an increase in hygiene, reduction of human interaction, and minimal use of artefacts in order to decrease the risk of virus transfer. Settings scaled down the range of choices for children and compartmentalised items for access by each bubble group. The resources and learning environment were sterilised after contact with every group of children. Two years later, these routines continue to be implemented in relation to the enduring nature of this pandemic and COVID guidance.

An unexpected outcome of this presentation of learning materials was an increase in the imaginative and creative play of children. The children used the limited resources to achieve a deeper level of learning by repeatedly exploring concepts over time and problem-solving by using materials for different functions. It was also observed that children were initiating interactive play more frequently with their peers, and they developed greater comprehension of sharing and turn-taking. It appeared that fewer external choices prompted the children to access implicit memories, leading to an increase in motivation, creativity, and group interactions. These anecdotal findings are important to consider, and current research is ongoing to explore the effect of COVID-19 upon education and care in the early years of childhood (Moore & Churchill, 2020).

Loose parts and divergent thinking

Outdoors is a rich natural environment that can be presented safely to children in services by eliminating the use of potentially dangerous areas and by creating a designated space for active play. The outdoor environment provides an extended opportunity for children to apply the skills achieved within heuristic play sessions. Play in a context of the natural world has a therapeutic effect due to the space, colours, sensory stimulation, freedom from human-made boundaries, and reduced social rules (Whitters, 2020). Divergent thinking is an aspect of development that is supported easily outdoors and evolves through scaffolding of play, role-modelling, prompting, creativity, and use of imagination.

Outdoor spaces have become invaluable resources which have gained significance within the context of COVID-19. Gardens and local woodland areas have rapidly been granted registration as safe play spaces in order to reduce numbers of children who play together inside and to present an environment which is deemed to minimise spread of this virus. It is 50 years since Nicholson (1971) published his theory on loose parts, and this pedagogical approach to educating children has become popular in recent years, with renewed interest during the pandemic of 2019 due to the outdoor context.

Nicholson (1971) placed emphasis on the role of practitioner in providing children with adequate choices and environments in which to learn, including indoors, outdoors, natural, and human-made resources. The rationale is to support development through opportunities for divergent thinking that nurture ability, capacity, and creativity. The adult observer is present as an attachment figure, but he does not interfere with the child's *play flow* and refrains from making suggestions, introducing ideas, or correcting actions. The atmosphere is quiet and conducive to the use of problem-solving and creativity through divergent thinking. This approach continues to be applied within services, and it is commonly encompassed within child-led pedagogy.

Play cycle

The play cycle refers to the processes that occur during play and include the play flow (King & Sturrock, 2020). The child expresses play cues externally which are based upon internal influences in relation to his interests, needs, and emotions. These play cues may also be given direction or prompts from another person or the proximal environment. The research findings by King and Sturrock (2020) indicated that play cues would reduce over time unless strengthened by interactions with another child or adult or an aspect of the environment. The distal environment can also affect the direction of play cues through sensory stimulation which links to familiar concepts. For example, the distant sound of an emergency vehicle's siren can induce specific cues, and it can inform imaginative actions.

The child's knowledge and understanding that is gained from interaction between his play cue and another person or environmental stimulus is termed the "play return". During observations by key workers, and analysis of each child's play, it can be useful to consider the source of the play return from a behavioural, environmental, or social cue. The play return is processed by the child who chooses to extend the play or to introduce another play cue; thus, a play cycle is completed (King & Sturrock, 2020).

There are six elements to a play cycle as termed by King and Sturrock (2020): metalude, play cue, play return, play frame, loop and flow, and annihilation. The metalude refers to the child's drive to participate in play. Internal influences result in his external expression through a play cue of actions and potentially words. If a response is not readily available to activate his play cue to a subsequent stage of the play cycle, then the child may issue a second cue, withdraw from play, or react with negative emotion (annihilation). If a response is available (play return), then a play frame is created. This frame may encompass physical and psychological elements. The play frame contributes to the child's learning and induces an increase in knowledge, understanding, and experiential learning. Developmental outcomes are gained through reciprocal interaction of the child's play cues and person or environmental feedback. These aspects inform the inner working model of the child and encompass the loop and flow stage of the play cycle. Play cues and returns will continue unless the child withdraws or this particular cycle is ended by another person or factor in the environment or social boundary.

The adult's role and responsibilities within a play cycle should be adapted to enrich the capacity and abilities of every child, and the ultimate outcome is a high level of well-being and involvement with a learning environment. For example, a practitioner may introduce a play cue to a child through role-modelling and support interpretation of an environment, particularly in contexts which are unfamiliar. During delivery of a therapeutic intervention (Bratton et al., 2006), I have found that children who have experienced trauma often require play cues to be introduced by the facilitator before participation in this context can commence. The important factor is the outcome of encouraging play and learning.

King and Sturrock (2020) commented upon this phenomenon within an investigation on cues for playful behaviour in an adult organisational meeting. Potential cues were provided on a material level by the use of objects and sweets which were displayed openly to employees within the environmental context. Findings indicated that these artefacts were associated with light-hearted behaviour from the adults in the meeting and regarded as cues or stimulation that led to frivolous behaviour in this particular context.

The play frame in services occurs within contexts that reflect social boundaries, health, and safety requirements, and respond to additional support for learning needs. It is necessary that the practitioner has a responsibility to have a "holding" role in the play frame. King and Sturrock (2020) applied this term within a discussion of data from a study in the UK. The research focused upon children's behaviour and practitioners' interpretation of play cues (Nottingham City Council & Russell, 2006). Findings had indicated that playworkers often misinterpreted play cues as challenging behaviour. The study concluded that adults have a role to play in maintaining the play frame in accordance with social and safety boundaries relevant to each setting and to the needs of each child. A description of containment was given by the authors to represent the adult role in supporting a child to adapt his play frame as necessary but to maintain the integrity of the child's original plan.

Containment involves the use of a broad skill set by a practitioner or parent which includes observation, interpretation, emotional literacy, assessment of risk, awareness of the child's interests and needs, and, ultimately, responsive intervention. The adult creates a dyad with a child, and he may be allocated an active or passive role within the play cycle. It is often the case that an adult's role fluctuates throughout an interaction and encompasses tentative steps by the adult and responsive, prompt reaction to the child's communications.

In 2020, research was conducted that reviewed the understanding of practitioners regarding the play cycle (King & Newstead, 2020). Findings indicated that comprehension was dependent on the source of practitioner's knowledge of this cycle and experience in the field. The use of pre-cue as explanatory for the term "metalude" has been inserted into the discussion by these authors, and it supports comprehension of the complex processes for practitioners in the early years and primary sector.

Play flow

Csikszentmihalyi (1975) defined flow as a holistic sensation and associated this experience with focused involvement in learning. This researcher commented that the term "flow" refers to the consistent nature of a person's actions as interactions take place with an environment or other people. This autotelic experience is led by the person's motivation in a particular context which can be related to interests, emotions, curiosity, creativity, and a desire to gain knowledge and understanding.

There is a significant characteristic of flow which was originally identified by Csikszentmihalyi (1975) and currently features in practitioner guidance in the early years and play work. Continuation of the play flow does not need a reward which is external to the child. The motivation to continue this experiential learning is driven by the child's inner working model. Csikszentmihalyi (1990) believed that the function of consciousness is for the inner working model to support each person to make sense of the internal and external world through use of prior knowledge, understanding, and emotional reactions. Emotions lead interpretation and contribute to the formation of perceptions which may differ for each person. A lack of consciousness relates to an immature sense of self and a child leading his life through the use of instinct and reflexes.

The flow can be interrupted if the child reflects upon the context, reviews his capacity, and alters his plan. For example, a child may confidently commence climbing upwards upon a wall frame driven by his internal motivation which maintains his physical competence. However, if the child stops and considers the height, danger, and isolation, then these negative interpretations can affect or halt the play flow on a temporary or longer-term basis. A child's focus upon negative influences can lead to disorder in his inner working model which affects interpretation of the environment and reaction to stimuli. An external prompt in the form of encouragement and empowerment from another person can support the immersion back into the play flow. Csikszentmihalyi (1990) commented that individuals who achieve a flow experience, despite adversities, demonstrate intrinsic motivation and are not easily distracted by external influences.

A process that follows flow is differentiation, and integration takes place throughout the learning experience. The infant or young child has an increase in capability and skill, and his thoughts and actions are integrated by a specific focus. The ability to capitalise upon personal skills, in order to maximise outcomes, depends on a child's capacity, which relates to his mental health and emotional status. Comprehension of flow experience highlights the significance of infant mental health and the role of adults in supporting well-being.

Csikszentmihalyi (1990) described happiness in terms of a flow experience in which each person's skill set matched available learning opportunities. This researcher described inner happiness as pertaining to harmony with oneself as opposed to an individual gaining control over the environment or other people. An activity is autotelic and becomes intrinsically rewarding and independent of the social environment. This outcome may occur during a child's involvement with the environment and alongside his interactions towards a planned goal.

Several theorists felt that the sensation and outcome of enjoyment was characterised by the principle of novelty (Csikszentmihalyi, 1990; Magnusson & Stattin, 2006). Attention is captured by curiosity, and it is a determining factor in improving quality of experiences along the continuum of enjoyment. Csikszentmihalyi (1990) identified major components of enjoyment, and these aspects are used to evaluate and inform assessment of a child's well-being and involvement during intervention. The Leuven Involvement and Well-being Scales (Laevers, 1994) are commonly used to interpret, to understand, and to record these issues by practitioners. From the child's perspective these components include:

- Tasks which are achievable by a child using his skill set.
- Identifying clear goals.
- Gaining timely feedback from an attachment figure.
- Experiencing meaningful involvement with an environment that provides respite from everyday pressures.
- Recognising a sense of control within this environment.
- No requirement for an immediate assessment or concern for safety of self.
- An unusual interpretation of the concept of time. For example, the passing of minutes may feel like hours, or hours may feel like they have passed within the usual temporal experience of passing minutes.

Additionally, Csikszentmihalyi (1990) identified three sources of support which a human being can access to deal with stressful situations: social networks, prior experience and understanding, and personality. Daily lifestyles provide opportunities for infants to explore independently, to make autonomous decisions, and to experience freedom in investigation and achievement of self-appointed goals. It is important for all children to feel nurtured within safe environments which leads to activation of intrinsic motivation. The presence of an attachment figure is the key to providing a foundation and context for internal stimulation to flourish and to increase resilience to life's adversities over time. The rationale is for children to make choices based upon personal evaluation of an experience as opposed to choices based upon external influences, for example, peer pressure or attempting to satisfy the needs of an adult. Csikszentmihalyi concluded by emphasising the importance of integration, cooperation, and universal flow which allow for individuality to be expressed.

The flow theory by Csikszentmihalyi et al. (2018) can be used to understand the processes of learning within everyday life and to provide guidance for working with children. This theory includes the importance of teaching children to focus upon external stimulation and to minimise their danger responses to a proximal environment. Learned responses may reflect adverse childhood experiences and impact upon the child's attention, retention, production, and motivation.

Transitions

The movement from one learning environment to another is recognised as a significant stage in a young child's developmental pathway. Transitions are not solely based upon familiarisation with the new environments but should primarily consider relationships, the child's sense of self, and potential change within a new environment. The relationship is a transitional medium which is essential to promote good mental health during the integration period. The rationale for positive transitions is based upon the understanding that a child should be supported within a secure attachment relationship to leave one area and to enter a new area. His ability to engage with learning has to be maintained and to be enhanced by the new circumstances in order that the transition has a positive impact upon development. A positive or negative transition can affect a child's learning over a long period of time.

The key internal transition between age groups in a service marks an important stage of development, and it is managed in accordance with the personal needs and circumstances of each child. There are several aspects to consider during the transition period. The child's current, and receiving, key worker should commence the process by planning the transition period with parents, and colleagues, in response to the child's needs. The child's referral details are discussed, stage of development, and child's ability and capacity to engage with a learning environment. The care plan is reviewed and updated.

Each child's personal interests, preferred medium of learning, and preferences are shared between the appropriate staff members.

The transition is discussed with a parent in a context of information exchange and collaboration. It is important to remember that the parent is also experiencing a transition between relationships and environments. The child is supported to prepare for leaving his current playroom by the use of photographs, discussion, and joint interactions with the new key worker. The child is supported to integrate into the new playroom alongside the new key worker by using a personal photograph, welcome time, opportunities for small and large group activities, inside and outside, and experiencing snack time. Similar processes should be experienced by the transitioning parent. A key strategy is supporting a child and his parent together and to project a sense of belonging within the new environment through role identity and clear expectations. Parents are given regular updates during this time and encouraged to talk to their child about the transition.

Transitions incur a child coping with the loss of a familiar relationship and the creation of a new secure attachment relationship. Five areas of development need to be considered in a context of transitions between, and within services. Changes for the child are multiple during this period, and expectations within each area of development should be established alongside the relational support. The following information highlights five areas of development, expectations of skill sets, and support which is founded on the attachment relationship.

1 **Physical**: A new environment invariably requires a child to extend or adapt his gross and fine motor skills. For example, the transition from home to a birth-to-2-year playroom or to a 2–3-year playroom presents many physical challenges to the young child. Tables, chairs, bikes, slide, trampoline, and small toys for manipulation are a few examples of artefacts that require the child to develop a new skill set during engagement and interaction. A secure relationship can minimise emotional barriers to the child's engagement with unfamiliar physical activities and underpin role-modelling and scaffolding to encourage exploration.

2 **Social**: A new environment encompasses relationships with different adults and peers, in addition to new social rules and expectations associated with routines and play experiences. Understanding a child's interpretation and reaction to a social environment informs the practitioner's reflective responding skills which facilitates the child's adaptation and involvement.

3 **Communication**: The visual and auditory stimuli within a 2–3-year playroom are vastly different to the birth-to-2-year playroom and may appear overwhelming to a young child. Friezes on the walls, and displays on floors and descending from the ceilings are used to communicate knowledge. The uptake is dependent on a child's ability to interpret information in this format. Verbal communication can be challenging to process for

the young transitioning 2-year-old. He is presented with language from adults and peers in many different styles and levels of comprehension. The secure relationship is used to encourage communication in the child's own learning mode.

4   **Intellectual and cognitive**: Many choices of play items are presented to a child within a 2-to-3-year playroom. Accessing these artefacts requires the child to interpret the social rules of play within child-led pedagogy. A secure relationship can be used to guide the child's involvement in the initial stages of transition and to create links to his previous learning environment. Transition toys may be used to create consistency between one environment and another and to create a familiar play experience for a child.

5   **Emotional**: Behaviour exhibits a child's knowledge of his world, interpretation at a particular point in time, and his associated emotions. Desire and motivation to learn are instinctive and activated in a context of emotional well-being but hindered by anxiety and stress. The child's stress should be managed responsively during a transition period. Social behaviour may be demonstrated at a lower level of development during the process of transferring from one learning environment to another, as a child seeks to comprehend the new circumstances and expectations. A child under duress may regress to display immature behaviours that reflect influences from previous childhood adversities.

Adversities may have a greater impact during transitions as the child's resilience to change can be lowered if he feels vulnerable and he has an increased level of anxiety. Interactions may indicate immaturity in development within the initial transition period. The relationship with a familiar adult is invaluable to promote emotional stability and mental health at this time; therefore, creation of secure attachment with a new key worker is significant to a positive transition.

Infant mental health: research, theory, and intervention

This book has explored infant mental health and used theory to gain comprehension of learning processes. As I complete the final chapter, the COVID-19 pandemic has entered another period of invasion across our world and represents a significant adverse childhood experience (Moore & Churchill, 2020). In the findings of the UK Trauma Council (2020), mitigation of these effects requires training in trauma responses by the professionals who educate and care for children. All children have potentially been affected by the pandemic, and the challenges for early years and primary teachers have increased. However, the human instinct to learn and to achieve is strong, and it can transcend adversities if the young learner is encompassed within supportive and responsive relationships.

The Association of Infant Mental Health, UK (2021) identifies seven domains as areas in which knowledge, comprehension, and practice should be developed:

1   Relationship-based practice.
2   Normal and atypical development.
3   Factors that influence caregiving capacity.
4   Assessment of caregiving.
5   Supporting caregiving.
6   Reflective practice and supervision.
7   Working within relevant legal and professional frameworks.

In a professional role, it is essential that reflection on competency considers any local or specific disciplinary parameters of knowledge and skills for use within practice. Experience cannot always be tagged neatly or easily to competency outcomes from a framework. It is often the case that formal support and supervision, and informal comments from colleagues or service-users, are the key to realisation of your own ability and capacity to achieve such outcomes.

It is widely acknowledged that practice strategies for generic teaching, or within a context of high ability, or responses to children with mental-health issues, are transferrable to all learners. Walsh et al. (2010) advised that a curriculum should be matched to the child's abilities and applied the term "developmentally appropriate curriculum". In order to implement curricula effectively within an early years services, the educator needs to understand the individuality of every child in his care. Educational contexts of inclusion and equality require teachers and early years practitioners to observe, to understand, and to respond to a child's engagement and well-being within a learning environment. Comprehension goes beyond the child's daily interactions, and it pays heed to direct and indirect influences in the form of adverse childhood experiences and protective factors in the home and community.

Educators, researchers, practitioners, and parents would agree that achievement of potential should be supported and promoted as appropriate to a child's capacity and interests. Observing and understanding a child's emotions, nurturing a secure attachment relationship, and facilitating involvement are key aspects which every educator should strive to achieve. Future practice is dependent on supporting professionals and carers to notice and to value each child's interactions, and, importantly, to nurture personal attainment and fulfilment.

A professional-to-parent helping relationship is formed in a context of unmet needs and a practitioner's desire and responsibility to respond by minimising the impact of adversities. These negative influences may be historical or current. Rogers (1990) described activation of the latent inner resources of a person who is seeking help through a supportive relationship. This researcher also highlighted a focus upon the sense of self and others during interactions. Rogers felt that awareness of the inner self created a healing presence within a dyad, which he identified as a transcendent phenomenon. As the developing person is changing then he is accompanied by the helper along an emotional journey which is constructed around a person-centred approach.

Rogers (1990) clarified his understanding of research and practice. The former provides a forum for reviewing a subjective topic with objectivity, and the latter provides the subjective experience. The practitioner may use research findings to extend his knowledge in an area in which he does not practice or to seek out further information on a particular topic of interest. Further education often leads educators towards research as a means to forging a career in an unfamiliar specialism.

Sigel (2006) reviewed the practitioner's need for research, and he identified an ability to absorb knowledge and to apply understanding to daily work as necessary steps in the transfer of research findings to practice in the field. The dissemination of research findings to the workforce may be sourced directly from the original research, the practitioner may be a participant in an investigation, or findings may inform local or national training and guidance.

Experiential learning provides practitioners with an essential first layer of applied knowledge. Our understanding is preliminary in the early stages. Over time, this interpretation becomes familiar, and we gain a sense of ownership and a right to be led by our emotions towards comprehension which is based upon professional skill. This emotional level is superficial, but familiarity with a concept over time, and opportunities to explore which are supported by research as a framework for learning, lead us towards a deeper understanding. Understanding has a subjective element which is based upon our lived experiences and interpretation influenced by prior learning. However, understanding also embraces an objective viewpoint which is informed by others and based upon their experiential learning and research. The outcome is a broad, rich construction that consolidates and transforms our inner working models.

I believe that each employer and employee has a responsibility to support the use of research in practice. O'Brien and Mitchell (2021) reported upon the valuable contribution of early years practitioners to a perinatal mental-health service in Sussex, England. Findings included knowledge of mental health from the early years participants and the experiences of services from the mothers' perspectives. The report concluded that practitioners were integrated positively into the mental-health team. Routes for each employee may vary and should accommodate the needs, abilities, and interests of practitioners. Practitioners who access generic guidance which is based upon research, practitioners as participants, or practitioner-researchers, provide rich sources of knowledge and understanding which are invaluable to developing practice in any workplace.

Final thoughts

I take time to reflect upon learning from my personal perspective as an early years practitioner and researcher in the twilight of my career. Reflection upon individual and collaborative practice is a common strategy which is applied on a daily basis to review and to develop implementation of a service and to justify funding for specific projects (Moon, 2004). Reflection on professional expertise and comprehension of a field are also mandatory aspects of registration by an appointed body, for example, Scottish Social Services Council (Scottish Social Services Council, 2003).

Reflective assessment is one aspect of a learning process that has to be judged against a standard in order to gain value and to contribute to a framework for development. Gibbs (1988) promotes a model of reflection which is used regularly by practitioners in care and education, at times inadvertently. The model encompasses review of current and past actions, and associated emotions. This approach is significant to my work context of child protection. Emotional impact can incentivise educators and support adherence to policy and procedure, or result in subjective judgement and create a dichotomy between professional and personal actions. It is essential to gain self-awareness during these processes.

Gaining sense and rationale for our actions is often achieved by consideration of emotions which can be influenced by our own childhood experiences, culture of a workplace, or mental health at a point in time. I have always used reflection for myself as a positive tool in recognising professional skill and areas for development. Each person learns from reflection of self and others. Actions are based upon teamwork, whether directly or indirectly. I feel that it is essential to widen the reflective scope beyond the individual and to consider the curtailing influences from strategic boundaries in addition to the freedom within operational skills of practice. I have learned over the years that strategy binds, and leads, or inhibits pedagogy and practice. However, practice without strategy and rationale may appear to liberate the practitioner but diminishes quality due to lack of boundaries and direction which can reduce consistency of a desired output.

The parent and infant form an interdependent dyad in the earliest stages of life which is influential throughout the lifespan. Effective professional–parent relationships are essential for the development of both generations and to enable sensitive interpretation and responses to needs, emotions, and mental health. The COVID-19 pandemic has resulted in many emotive conversations being conducted outside service buildings in cold, wet, and challenging environments. I feel humbled by the trust and respect which parents bestow upon teams. We have all quickly adapted to COVID-19 regulations, and strategies can be effective if responsive to need. It is important to notice, and to capitalise upon, help-seeking overtures from parents.

The pandemic has certainly increased professional understanding of empathic relationships and infant mental health. It is clear that the human need for relationships continues to be at the forefront of our daily existence. A therapeutic alliance can be created in any environment and can facilitate the learning and development of parent and child.

A study published in 2021 reviewed 40 family intervention programmes from the USA, Australia, UK, Sweden, Netherlands, Canada, Denmark,

Finland, and France (Lagdon et al., 2021). Findings indicated that 25–50 per cent of the children whose parents had a mental-health issue experienced a psychological disorder during childhood or adolescence. Subsequently, 10–14 per cent of these children received a diagnosis of psychotic disorder during childhood or adulthood. This study also links parental mental-health issues and child abuse, as published by previous authors (Cleaver et al., 2011; Finkelhor et al., 2015). The investigation concluded that a universal definition of family-focused practice would encapsulate key strategies and rationale. Additionally, despite a consistency of components across the 40 studies, and within each country, greater emphasis on engagement with local community supports was recommended by the authors.

Change which is embedded within a family and local community encompasses factors of sustainability, and positive long-term outcomes. A valid response to infant mental-health issues is joint working between adult mental-health services and children's services. Strengthening the links between research, theory, and practice, in a context of change and development of family units would upskill the workforce in this field. Researchers, practitioners, and parents are key contributors to supporting infant mental health.

References

Association of Infant Mental Health, UK. (2021). The infant mental health competency framework. https://aimh.uk/the-uk-imh-competency-framework.

Barlow, J. (2016). Improving attachment in babies: What works? Association of Infant Mental Health best practice guidance no.2. https://aimh.uk/news-resources/members-only-resources.

Benjamin, L. S., & Karpiak, C. P. (2001). Personality disorders. *Psychotherapy: Theory, Research, Practice, Training*, 38(4), 487–491. https://www.psycnet.apa.org/record/2002-01390-023.

Berlin, L. J., Zeanah, C. H., & Lieberman, A. F. (2008). Prevention and intervention programmes for supporting early attachment security. In J. Cassidy & P. R. Shaver (Eds.), *Handbook of attachment, theory, research, and clinical applications*, 2nd edition (pp. 745–761). New York: The Guilford Press.

Bowlby, J. (1997). *Attachment and loss*. London: Pimlico.

Bratton, S. C., Landreth, G. L., Kellam, T., & Blackard, S. R. (2006). *Child/parent participation therapy treatment manual*. New York: Routledge.

Braun, D., Davis, H., & Mansfield, P. (2006). *How helping works: Towards a shared model of process*. London: The Centre for Parent and Child Support.

Bretherton, I., & Munholland, K. A. (2008). Internal working models in attachment relationships, elaborating a central construct in attachment theory. In J. Cassidy & P. R. Shaver (Eds.), *Handbook of attachment, theory, research, and clinical applications*, 2nd edition (pp. 102–127). New York: The Guilford Press.

Bronfenbrenner, U. (1979). *The ecology of human development*, 2nd edition. Cambridge, MA: Harvard University Press.

Bronfenbrenner, U. (2005). *Making human beings human, biological perspectives on human development*. Thousand Oaks, CA: Sage.

Bronfenbrenner, U., & Morris, P. A. (2006). The bioecological model of human development. In W. Damon & R. M. Lerner (Eds.), *Handbook of child psychology*, vol. I. Hoboken, NJ: Wiley & Sons.

Cain, D. J. (2010). *Person-centred psychotherapies*. Washington, DC: American Psychological Association.

Cleaver, H., & Freeman, P. (1995). *Parental perspectives in cases of suspected child abuse*. London: Her Majesty's Stationery Office.

Cleaver, H., Unell, I., & Aldgate, J. (2011). *Children's needs – parenting capacity: Child abuse – parental mental illness, learning disability, substance misuse, and domestic violence*. London: TSO.

Clemens, V., Berthold, O., Witt, A., Brahler, E., Plener, P. L., & Fegert, J. M. (2020). Childhood adversities and later attitudes towards harmful parenting behaviour including shaking in a German population-based sample. *Child Abuse Review*, 29, 269–281.

Csikszentmihalyi, M. (1975). *Beyond boredom and anxiety: The experience of play in work and games*. San Francisco, CA: Josey-Bass Inc. Publishers.

Csikszentmihalyi, M. (1990). *Flow: The psychology of experience*. New York: HarperCollins.

Csikszentmihalyi, M., Montijo, M. N., & Mouton, A. R. (2018). Flow theory: optimising elite performance in the creative realm. In S. I. Pfeiffer (Ed.), *APA handbook of giftedness and talent* (pp. 215–229). Washington, DC: American Psychological Association.

Doyle, C., & Cicchetti, D. (2017). From the cradle to the grave: The effect of adverse caregiving environments on attachment and relationships throughout the lifespan institute of child development. *Clinical Psychology, Science, and Practice*, 24, 203–217.

Duffy, M., Walsh, C., Mulholland, C., Davidson, G., Best, P., Bunting, L., Herron, S., Quinn, P., Gillanders, C., Sheehan, C., & Devaney, J. (2021). Screening children with a history of maltreatment for PTSD in frontline social care organisations: An explorative study. *Child Abuse Review*, 30(6), 594–611.

Early Learning and Childcare Directorate. (2020). *Phase 1: Easing of lockdown in Scotland*. Edinburgh: Scottish Government.

Education Scotland. (2020). *A summary of resources relating to highly able learners*. Livingston: Education Scotland.

Finkelhor, D., Shattuck, A., Turner, H., & Hamby, S. (2015). A revised inventory of adverse childhood experiences. *Child Abuse and Neglect*, 48, 13–21. https://www.unh.edu/ccrc/pdf/CV334.pdf.

Gibbs, G. (1988). *Learning by doing: A guide to teaching and learning methods*. Oxford: Further Education Unit, Oxford Polytechnic.

Gross, J. J. (1999). Emotion and emotion regulation. In L. A. Pervin & O. P. Johns. (Eds.), *Handbook of personality: theory and research*, 2nd edition (pp. 525–552). New York: Guilford Press.

Hogg, S. (2019). *Rare jewels, specialised parent-infant relationship teams in the UK*. https://parentinfantfoundation.org.uk/wp-content/uploads/2019/09/PIPUK-Rare-Jewels-FINAL.pdf.

King, P., & Newstead, S. (2020). Re-defining the play cycle: An empirical study of playworkers' understanding of play-work theory. *Journal of Early Childhood Research*, 18(1), 99–111.

King, P., & Sturrock, G. (2020). *The play cycle: theory, research, and application*. Abingdon and New York: Routledge.

Klein, M. H., Kolden, G. G., Michels, J. L., & Chisholm-Stockard, S. (2002). Congruence. In J. C. Norcross (Ed.), *Psychotherapy relationships that work*. Oxford: Oxford University Press.

Laevers, F. (1994). *The project experiential education: Concepts and experiences at level of context, process, and outcome*. Leuven: Leuven University.

Lagdon, S., Grant, A., Davidson, G., Devaney, J., Donaghy, M., Duffy, J., Galway, K., & McCartan, C. (2021). Families with parental mental health problems: A systematic narrative review of family-focused practice. *Child Abuse Review*, 30(5), 400–421.

Lave, J., & Wenger, E. (1991). *Situated learning, legitimate peripheral participation*. Cambridge: Cambridge University Press.

Lazarus, R. S. (1991). *Emotion and adaptation*. Oxford: Oxford University Press.

Magnusson, D., & Stattin, H. (2006). The person in context: A holistic-interactionist approach. In W. Damon & R. Lerner (Eds.), *Handbook of child psychology*, vol. I. Hoboken, NJ: John Wiley & Sons.

Mikulincer, M., & Shaver, P. R. (2008). Adult attachment and affect regulation. In J. Cassidy & P. R. Shaver (Eds.), *Handbook of attachment, theory, research, and clinical applications*, 2nd edition (pp. 503–531). New York: The Guilford Press.

Moon J. A. (2004). A handbook of reflective and experiential learning: theory and practice. London: Routledge

Moore, E., & Churchill, G. (2020). Still here for children: Experiences of NSPCC staff who supported children and families during COVID-19. https://learning.nspcc.org.uk/research-resources/2020/still-here-for-children-experiences-of-nspcc-staff-during-coronavirus.

Moran, P., Ghate, D., & van der Merwe, A. (2004). *What works in parenting support? A review of the international evidence*. London: Department for Education and Skills.

Nagy, A. V. & Nagy, V. (2022). A SARS COVID-19 vírus okozta helyzet a hazai kora gyermekkori intézményekben [The effect of SARS-COVID-19 virus in Early Childhood Education in Hungary]. https://www.researchgate.net/publication/357661708_A_SARS_COVID-19_VIRUS_OKOZTA_HELYZET_A_HAZAI_KORA_GYER MEKKORI_INTEZMENYEKBEN_The_Effect_of_SARS-COVID-19_VIRUS_in_Early_Childhood_Education_in_Hungary.

National Scientific Council on the Developing Child. (2020). Connecting the brain to the rest of the body: Early childhood development and lifelong health are deeply intertwined. Working paper no. 15. https://developingchild.harvard.edu/resources/connecting-the-brain-to-the-rest-of-the-body-early-childhood-development-and-life long-health-are-deeply-intertwined.

Nicholson, S. (1971). How not to cheat children: The theory of loose parts. *Landscape Architecture*, 62(1), 30–34.

Nottingham City Council & Russell, W. (2006). *Play-work impact evaluation: Final report*. Nottingham: Nottingham City Council.

O'Brien, R., & Mitchell, C. (2021). The role of early years practitioners in a perinatal mental health service. *International Journal of Birth and Parent Education* 9(1), 33–36. https://www.ijbpe.com/journals/volume-9/57-vol-9-issue-1

Rogers, C. (1990). Speaking personally. In H. Kirschenbaum & V. L. Henderson (Eds.), *The Carl Rogers reader* (p. 16). London: Constable.

Ryecraft, J. R. (2019). Behind the walls of poverty: Economically disadvantaged gifted and talented children. In J. T. Pardeck & J. W. Murphy (Eds.), *Young gifted children, identification, programming, and socio-psychological issue* (pp. 139–147). Abingdon: Routledge.

Scottish Government. (2009). *Changing lives*. Edinburgh: Scottish Government.

Scottish Government. (2021). Child neglect in Scotland: Understanding causes and supporting families, child protection committees, Scotland, October 2021. https://www.gov.scot/publications/national-guidance-child-protection-scotland-2021.

Scottish Social Services Council. (2003). *Codes of practice for social services workers and employers, code* 1. Dundee: Scottish Social Services Council.

Sigel, I. E. (2006). Research to practice redefined. In W. Damon & R. Lerner (Eds.), *Handbook of child psychology, child psychology in practice*, vol. IV, 6th edition (pp. 1017–1023). Hoboken, NJ: John Wiley & Sons.

Simpson, J. A., & Belsky, J. (2008). Attachment theory within a modern evolutionary framework. In J. Cassidy & P. R. Shaver (Eds.), *Handbook of attachment, theory, research, and clinical applications*. 2nd edition (pp. 131–157). New York: The Guilford Press.

Spencer, M. B. (2006). Phenomenology and ecological systems theory: Development of diverse groups. In R. M. Lerner & W. Damon (Eds.), *Handbook of child psychology: Theoretical models of human development* (pp. 829–893). Hoboken, NJ: John Wiley & Sons.

Tal, C. (2021). An ecosystem perspective of practice and professional development in early childhood education and care (ECEC). *European Early Childhood Education Research Journal*, 29(6), 809–812.

Taylor, I. (2019). We need to talk about differentiation in schools. *TES Magazine*, 8 November. https://www.tes.com/magazine/article/we-need-talk-about-differentiation-schools.

Thelen, E., & Smith, L. B. (2006). Dynamic systems theory. In W. Damon & R. Lerner (Eds.), *Handbook of child psychology*, vol. I (pp. 258–312). Hoboken, NJ: John Wiley & Sons.

Thompson, R. A. (2008). Early attachment and later development, familiar questions, new answers. In J. Cassidy & P. R. Shaver (Eds.), *Handbook of attachment, theory, research, and clinical applications*, 2nd edition (pp. 348–365). New York: The Guilford Press.

Trotter, C. (2002). Worker skill and client outcome in child protection. *Child Abuse Review*, 11, pp. 38–50.

UK Trauma Council. (2020). Beyond the pandemic: Strategic priorities for responding to childhood trauma. A coronavirus pandemic policy briefing. https://uktraumacouncil.org/wp-content/uploads/2020/09/Coronavirus-CYP-and-Trauma-UKTC-Policy-Briefing-Sept-2020.pdf.

Walsh, R. L., Hodge, K. A., Bowes, J. M., & Kemp, C. R. (2010). Same age, different page: overcoming the barriers to catering for young, gifted children in prior-to-school settings. *International Journal of Early Childhood*, 42(1), 43–58.

Whitters, H. G. (2015). Perceptions of the influences upon the parent-professional relationship in a context of early intervention and child protection. Ph.D. thesis. University of Strathclyde.

Whitters, H. G. (2017). *Nursery nurse to early years' practitioner: Role, relationships and responsibilities*. Abingdon: Oxford.

Whitters, H. G. (2020). *Adverse childhood experiences, attachment, and the early years' learning environment, research, and inclusive practice*. Abingdon and New York: Routledge.

Zero to Three (2017). The basics of infant and early childhood mental health: A briefing paper. https://www.zerotothree.org/policy-and-advocacy/social-and-emotional-health.

Zhou, M., & Brown, D. (2015). *Educational learning theories*, 2nd edition, Education Open Textbooks, 1. https://oer.galileo.usg.edu/education-textbooks/1.

Index